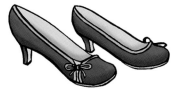

CLOSET CONFIDENTIAL

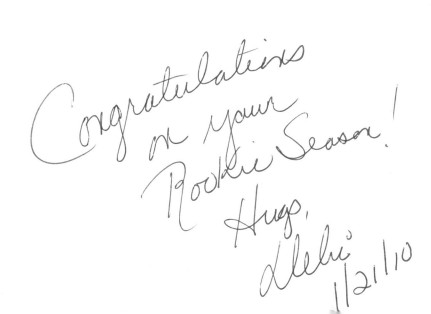

Congratulations on your Rookie Season!

Hugs,

Llebi

1/21/10

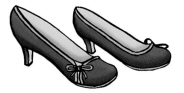

CLOSET CONFIDENTIAL
(STYLE SECRETS LEARNED <u>THE</u> HARD WAY)
WINONA DIMEO-EDIGER

Illustrations by Sam Trout

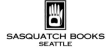

SASQUATCH BOOKS
SEATTLE

For every woman who's ever
had a full closet and nothing to wear.

Also, my mom.

Printed in China

Published by Sasquatch Books
Distributed by PGW/Perseus

15 14 13 12 11 10 09   9 8 7 6 5 4 3 2 1

COVER AND INTERIOR DESIGN: Lesley Feldman
COVER ILLUSTRATIONS: Sam Trout
INTERIOR COMPOSITION: Lesley Feldman / Liza Brice-Dahmen
INTERIOR ILLUSTRATIONS: Sam Trout and Winona Dimeo-Ediger
INTERIOR MAP: © Antuanas | Dreamstime.com
AUTHOR PHOTO: Winona Dimeo-Ediger

Library of Congress Cataloging-in-Publication Data

Dimeo-Ediger, Winona.

  Closet confidential : style secrets learned the hard way / Winona Dimeo-
Ediger ; illustrations by Sam Trout.

       p. cm.

  Includes index.

  ISBN-13: 978-1-57061-615-0

  ISBN-10: 1-57061-615-9

  1. Clothing and dress. 2. Clothing and dress--Humor. 3. Fashion--Humor. I.
Title.

  TT507.D55 2009

  646.4002'07--dc22

                        2009017767

SASQUATCH BOOKS
119 South Main Street, Suite 400
Seattle, WA 98104
(206) 467-4300

www.sasquatchbooks.com
custserv@sasquatchbooks.com

CONTENTS

Acknowledgments

There is a page in my seventh grade journal that looks like this:

People to thank when I write a book:

1. *The Backstreet Boys*
2. *Ms. Blackman*

So I guess that's a good place to start. I'd like to thank the Backstreet Boys, especially AJ, and Ms. Blackman, my seventh grade social studies teacher.

Other, more minor players who deserve my thanks: Sara Freedman, my amazing developmental editor, without whose humor and guidance this book would simply not exist; and Terence Maikels and everyone at Sasquatch Books for their talent, kindness, and genuine enthusiasm for this project.

Paul Collins is as good a person as he is a writer, and I am so grateful for his support, advice, and literary street cred. Vicki Ballou could have charged me $1,000,000 for all the assistance she gave me, but she did it for free.

Thank you to my family for making sure I never run out of material (and Tona, specifically, for gathering mule facts). Thank you to my friends for sharing their stories and squeals of excitement. Thank you to Nick for always believing in me.

Most of all, I want to thank my fellow fashion bloggers and the wonderful readers of Daddy Likey. This online community of smart, stylish women and men from around the world gives me endless inspiration and encouragement.

Introduction

One day, you open up a fashion magazine and it says, in bold block letters:

WIDE-LEG TROUSERS ARE A CLASSIC! WEAR THEM EVERY DAY! YOU CAN'T GO WRONG!

A week later, you're watching a makeover show on TV and see the hosts rip a pair of pants from a crying woman, scolding, "Wide-leg trousers are SO five years ago! What are you thinking?"

You consider joining a nudist colony. I don't blame you.

Style rules tend to be harsh and confusing, which is why this is not a book about style rules. In *Closet Confidential*, you'll find fashion tips, ideas, stories, and, most importantly, fifty style lessons straight from my cache of personal experiences/humiliations. I once constructed a turban out of an old pair of jeans and wore it to class, so I'm not one to cast style rule stones.

I've always been into fashion (as a child I favored customized puff paint T-shirts and neon leggings), but I haven't always been into how the fashion world operates—unapproachable, expensive, and steadfastly size 2 are among my least favorite adjectives. I started my fashion blog Daddy Likey (daddylikey.blogspot.com) because I wanted to create a place where style, smarts, and self-deprecation could finally coexist. Plus, I wanted to write haiku about ugly jumpsuits, but that was a secondary motivation.

This is a book for real women with real bodies and real budgets and a real desire to carve out their own personal style. Fashion is fun. Don't let any other book or magazine or TV show or cynical friend convince you otherwise. Have fun with this book and have fun getting dressed every day.

Learn from my fashion mistakes, but don't be afraid to make your own.

ONE

The Definitive Guide to Shopping for Jeans While Retaining at Least One-Third of Your Self-Esteem

(AND AT LEAST ONE-HALF OF YOUR PAYCHECK)

MY MOM TOOK ME SHOPPING for my first pair of jeans when I was twelve years old. I was a chubby child and up until then, I had favored elastic-waisted leggings and cotton-Lycra skorts. The day we set out to begin this new chapter of my life, I was ecstatic. I couldn't wait to slip on a perfect pair of jeans and transform into one of the cool, casual, all-American girls I saw on TV. I envisioned folding my crisp indigo jeans and gingerly placing them in my purple dresser, next to my compass and crime-fighting notebook, while whispering things like, "We've done it again, Old Blue," and "I can't wait for the adventures tomorrow will bring!"

By the time we finally arrived at the mall, I had worked myself into a denim-fueled hysteria. I was, perhaps, the most enthusiastic and delusional customer that Gap had ever seen.

But my eager young self was soon hit with the harsh realities of life in the real world: unflattering dressing room lighting, a salesclerk who seemed unfamiliar with the definition of tact ("hmm . . . your waist is much bigger than I thought"), and an intimidating and confusing array of styles and colors. I left the store with a pair of saggy, tapered jeans and a maxim that has stuck with me to adulthood—shopping for jeans is hell.

Jeans are made out to be the great equalizer, the easy, comfy, throw-'em-on, be-all-end-all style solution, when in fact, they're just pants made out of denim, and a well-fitting pair of pants is hard to find. Everyone knows that shopping for, say, a swimsuit is going to be a miserable experience, so they go in adequately prepared (or intoxicated). We must exercise this same vigilance when jeans shopping so that the difficulties do not take us by surprise.

Prepare for jeans shopping the same way you'd prepare for rigorous samurai training: plan out a block of time, be knowledgeable about the task at hand, visualize success, and know that the sweat and tears are totally worth it.

JEANS SHOPPING 101

➤ **PLAN AHEAD.** For example, don't schedule your shopping trip right after your dinner at the pasta buffet. Leave plenty of time to peruse the store. Pack a flask and rescue flares in case things get really bad.

➤ **KNOW EXACTLY WHAT KIND OF JEANS YOU'RE SHOPPING FOR** and dress accordingly. If you're looking for relaxed everyday jeans, wear casual shoes, shirt, and undergarments. If you're searching for some trendier denim to wear with heels at night, then wear your stilettos and a clingy top to the store. Want a pair of skinny jeans to tuck into your boots? Wear your boots into the dressing room and tuck those jeans in.

➤ **KEEP A BALLPARK PRICE IN MIND.** And no, $20–$200 is not a ballpark. Is this going to be a sale rack kind of day, or is this going to be the day you spend some (or all) of your savings on a pair of designer jeans?

➤ **IF YOU USUALLY HAVE A HARD TIME FINDING JEANS,** steer clear of smaller stores and boutiques, and head straight for large stores with larger selections. There's nothing worse than trying on every single pair of jeans in a store only to go home empty-handed, convinced you're some kind of mutant who can't wear normal clothes, when in fact, the store only offered three different styles.

➤ **IF YOU HAVE A LITTLE JUNK IN THE TRUNK** or have been blessed with a Rubenesque figure, you should check out stores that specialize in larger sizes—they usually have more options, and the staff has a better knowledge of flattering cuts and colors.

➤ **CONVERSELY, IF YOU HAVE A SMALLER FRAME,** or are just looking for a bargain, don't be afraid to take a peek at the juniors' section, especially for trendier styles. Prices usually stay below $50, but beware the super-low-rise fashions, which only tend to look good on svelte thirteen-year-olds.

➤ **AS MUCH AS I ADORE THRIFT AND VINTAGE STORES,** they are not dependable sources for jeans. If you stumble across a fabulous pair of worn-in Levi's while browsing at the thrift store, good for you. But usually, the selection is too limited and unpredictable to count on finding a good fit.

➤ **NO MATTER WHAT STORE YOU GO TO,** try on five hundred pairs of jeans . . . and then try on five more. Do you see why you should carve out some time for this?

➤ **IF YOU HYPERVENTILATE** at the thought of endless shelves of denim, familiarize yourself with the Denim Field Guide and Maslow's Hierarchy of Jeans (both coming up later in this chapter) to help you make sense of it all. You could breathe into a paper bag too, if that helps.

Finding the Style for You

A long time ago, probably in the sixteenth century, a prominent clothier proclaimed that all women look good in boot cut jeans. Oprah and makeover shows followed suit, and soon many of us had become staunch boot cut loyalists. While boot cut jeans are indeed quite flattering, there's a big, bright world of denim out there that gets overlooked when we always reach for the boot cuts.

Until about a year ago, I was a card-carrying member of the Boot Cut Legion. I wore dark wash boot cut jeans every day, and when I went shopping for jeans, I bought more dark wash boot cut jeans, and I felt pretty good about it. Then, while browsing department store sale racks one day, I saw the jeans that would change my life: they were slim fitting, straight legged, and cropped at the ankle. They had badass '80s zippers at the hems and fading on the thighs. They were everything that a short girl with generous thighs is trained to flee from and never look back at, but I couldn't look away.

I tried them on, and they were seriously amazing. The cropped length somehow looked charming on my stubby legs, and when paired with ballet flats and a cute sweater, the effect was very punk rock Jackie O. They were so much more me than any of the bland boot cut jeans in my denim wardrobe, and I ended up buying two pairs of my new find.

The constitution guarantees freedom of speech, press, religion, petition, assembly, and to wear any style of jeans we want, so try something new— you might be pleasantly surprised.

Ask any woman on the street what kind of jeans she is *supposed* to wear, and she probably won't miss a beat before robotically reciting, "I balance out my large hips with a flared leg," "My boyish frame requires a low-rise boot cut style," or "Why the hell are you asking me this? Do I know you?"

Knowing what type of jeans work for you can be a wonderful asset, but it can also get you stuck in a rut, frozen with fear at the mere prospect of trying a different color or slightly slimmer or wider legs.

Here's my suggestion: Go to the store and try on a few styles you never thought you could wear. Don't be intimidated by skinny styles or giant bell bottoms, even if every magazine and every salesgirl and every other fashion book says, "No, no, no, don't do it!" Sure, the jeans might look shockingly bad (that's why you packed a flask), but they might look shockingly good, too. Who knows what you've been missing?

If you come away knowing that boot cut really is the best style for you, then rock those boot cuts, girlfriend. And if you discover that a certain pair of skinny jeans does wonders for your voluptuous curves, more power to you. But you'll never know until you try.

DENIM FIELD GUIDE

Boot Cut Jeans

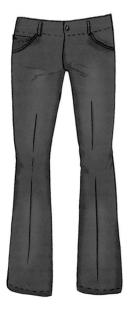

boot cut jeans

Latin Name: *Jeanus versatilus*

General Description: The boot cut style is a straight leg with a slight flare at the bottom. It is quite handy to wear with boots.

Habitat: This style of jean is massively popular and can be observed on a wide variety of individuals, from soccer moms to college students.

Range: A great choice for everyday wear and weekend outings; the darker-colored varieties work for some office environments or out on the town.

Mates (Northern): Tank tops, T-shirts, blazers, jackets, tunics.

Mates (Southern): Boots, flats, low- and mid-height wedges.

Natural Enemies: Super–high heels.

Summary of Behavior and Discussion: The boot cut jean is versatile and flattering on most body types, although its proliferation has made it a bit of a style snore. Still, boot cut is a good standby that will rarely let you down.

Straight Leg Jeans

Latin Name: *Jeanus versatilus II*

General Description: Straight leg jeans are a close cousin of boot cut jeans, different only in that the former lacks the slight flare, maintaining a straight line down the leg from waist to ankle. Straight leg jeans can be slim fitting, to the point of resembling a skinny jean, or baggier.

Habitat: See boot cut.

Range: See boot cut.

Mates (Northern): Tank tops, T-shirts, blazers, jackets, tunics.

Mates (Southern): Flats, wedges, heels, boots.

Summary of Behavior and Discussion: Straight leg jeans don't get as much love as boot cut but can be just as flattering. I'm a huge fan.

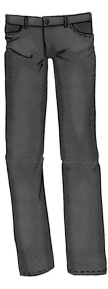

straight leg jeans

Skinny Jeans

Latin Name: *Extreme intimidatus*

General Description: This close-fitting jean fits tightly all the way down the leg to a tapered opening at the ankle.

Habitat: Commonly found on Hollywood starlets, Emo boys, hipsters, skinny teenage girls, and a number of brave, nonskinny women.

Range: Skinny jeans are most at home in casual environments, although they can be pushed toward formality with a cute top and high heels.

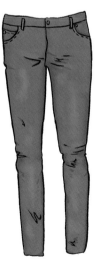

skinny jeans

Mates (Northern): To offset their teeny-tiny proportions, best with tunic tops, flowy shirts, and oversized cardigans.

Mates (Southern): Extraordinarily cute with pointy-toed flats or thick high heels. The best jeans for tucking into boots, since the legs won't bunch.

Summary of Behavior and Discussion: Despite their extremely intimidating moniker, these creatures are not as evil as they look. They can be a wonderful tool to keep in your wardrobe (even if you're not "skinny") for balancing out voluminous tops or tucking into boots, and different colors and lengths can be surprisingly flattering. Seriously, try 'em out. I'll give you a dollar.

Flare Jeans

Latin Name: *Disco throwbackus*

General Description: The opposite of a tapered leg, flares encompass any jeans with flared leg openings larger than those on boot cuts, all the way up to and including giant bell bottoms.

Habitat: Exaggerated flare styles are popular with teenagers and people who might argue with the statement "Jerry Garcia is dead." Smaller flares are super cute and look good on most people.

Range: Jeans with flares larger than those on boot cuts are usually a little too trendy for an office (of course, it always depends on the office), but they're wonderful for nights out and weekends.

Mates (Northern): Slim-fitting tops, blazers, cardigans, hoodies.

Mates (Southern): Anything with a thick heel to balance out the volume of the flare—platforms and wedges are great.

Summary of Behavior and Discussion: The flare jean is an excellent option for those who want to try something a little different from a boot cut, but not too different. More fun and trendy than boot cuts, flares command the same power to balance out larger hips and thighs. What's not to love?

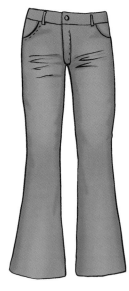

flare jeans

Mom Jeans

Latin Name: *Don't go there. Seriouslyus.*

General Description: Shares the tapered leg seen on skinny jeans, but mom jeans often lack flattering stretch, are light colored, and bunch and sag around the crotch.

Habitat: Alas, the proverbial "mom."

Range: Most common in the suburban United States and "before" photos on makeover television shows.

Mates (Northern): Frequently seen with baggy T-shirts and stained alma mater sweatshirts.

Mates (Southern): Dirty sneakers, flip-flops.

Summary of Behavior and Discussion: These sartorial pests are the bane of makeover show hosts around the globe, and for good reason: mom jeans don't look good on anyone. While there is a fine line between the mom jean and the skinny jean, it is an important line that is dangerous to cross.

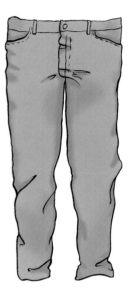

mom jeans

High-Waisted Jeans

Latin Name: *Crotch infinitus*

General Description: Jeans with a high rise that hits just above the belly button or, in extreme cases, just under your boobs.

Habitat: Pop stars, daring fashionistas, and resourceful women who know how to use these jeans' stomach-sucking power for good.

Range: High-waisted jeans usually look more formal than their low-rise counterparts; dark denim versions are acceptable wherever normal work trousers can go.

Mates (Northern): For a full Love Boat vibe, try a tucked-in ruffle-necked shirt, peacoat, and silk scarf.

Mates (Southern): Heels, platforms, wedges, boots (anything with a heel—it's good to elongate the legs to match the elongated rise of the jean).

Natural Enemies: High-rise skinny jeans rarely do anyone any favors.

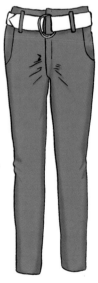

high-waisted jeans

Summary of Behavior and Discussion: High-waisted jeans are an excellent option for fashion daredevils and those craving a throwback to '70s glamour. Additionally, flat-front high-waisted jeans are the secret weapon of those looking for nothing more than a little tummy control: as a friend of mine once pointed out, "If you don't tuck in your shirt, they're just a girdle."

Low-Rise Jeans

Latin Name: *Accidental exhibitionus*

General Description: Also known as hip-huggers, low-rise jeans sit low (like, really low) on the hips.

Habitat: 13-year-old girls and other people who should maybe reconsider (myself included).

Range: Casual environments such as classrooms, from middle school through college.

Mates (Northern): Wide belts, slim-fitting T-shirts, sweaters.

Mates (Southern): Often seen with plastic flip-flops.

Natural Enemies: Short shirts, exposed G-strings.

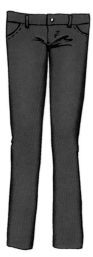

low-rise jeans

Summary of Behavior and Discussion: For most of my adolescence, I believed that since I was young and hip, I should wear low-rise jeans. I neglected to take into account my round gut and general discomfort with showing my butt to strangers. While the low-rise styles look good on some people, the day I discovered mid-rise jeans was a very good day indeed.

Cutoffs

Latin Name: *Jeanus interruptus*

General Description: Cutoffs begin their lives as any of the jeans mentioned here and become custom-length shorts.

Habitat: Carefree kids, hippies, and adorable women everywhere.

Range: Widespread during the summer months.

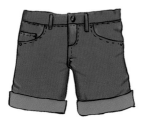

cutoffs

Mates (Northern): T-shirts, breezy plaid button-ups, tank tops.

Mates (Southern): Sneakers, flip-flops, sandals.

Summary of Behavior and Discussion: I tend to make a pair of cutoffs whenever I get too hot, so by the end of every summer, I don't have any more long pants. While I wouldn't recommend such extreme behavior, I do believe that cutoffs are a fun and functional wardrobe staple.

Denim Skirt

Latin Name: *Woman's best friendus*

General Description: The denim skirt is a piece that came into fashion in the '60s and hasn't gone out of style since.

Habitat: Denim miniskirts are often found on teenagers; knee-length denim skirts look good on everyone; floor-length denim skirts can be seen on gothic club kids and Mennonites.

Range: A denim skirt of a flattering length can take you from the mall to the movies to the potluck, and every casual event in between.

Mates (Northern): Where to begin? Chunky-knit sweaters, twinsets, T-shirts, hoodies.

Mates (Southern): Bright tights, kneesocks, pointy-toed flats, wedges, boots.

Natural Enemies: As a general rule, high heels and short skirts do not mix.

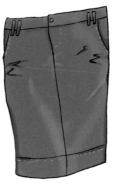

denim skirt

Summary of Behavior and Discussion: From sassy minis to floor-length styles, there's a denim skirt out there for everyone. Each makes for an excellent outfit base—add a T-shirt and sandals for a classic, simple look, or neon tights, a leather jacket, and boots for a funkier style.

Overalls

Latin Name: *Hick uniformus*

General Description: Ah, the humble overall, as American as apple pie! That is, if apple pie were made of denim and made everybody look pregnant.

Habitat: The denim overall thrives in farming communities, where it is the cliché uniform of choice. It is also popular among pregnant women, young starlets trying to make overalls trendy, and toddlers.

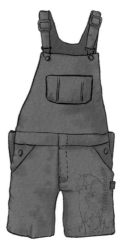

overalls

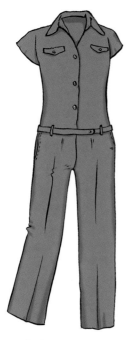

denim jumpsuit

Range: Appalachia. Preschools. The Gap maternity section. "Fashion Police" sections of tabloid magazines.

Summary of Behavior and Discussion: While overalls are usually unflattering, I LOVE THEM. There, I said it.

Denim Jumpsuits

Extinct.

BUILDING YOUR DENIM WARDROBE

Now that you have reviewed the Denim Field Guide, it's time to decide which styles of jeans have a place in your personal denim wardrobe. It's best to make sure you have your everyday necessities first, and then work your way up to some frivolous, fabulous options. Please consult the figure on the next page for more information.

Maslow's Hierarchy

Maslow's Heirarchy of Needs is a well-known psychological theory that illustrates, in a handy pyramid shape, five levels of human needs, beginning with our most basic needs at the bottom (food, shelter, sleep, sample sales, etc.) and building up to self-actualization (creativity, spontaneity, etc.) at the peak. Little did Ol' Man Maslow know that his theory also relates to jeans.

First (Bottom or Base) Row (Physiological, Basic Needs): Two pairs of well-fitting quality jeans in medium to dark wash that you feel comfortable and sexy in. Appropriate for activities ranging from work to school to dates to shopping.

Second Row (Safety): One to four pairs of schlepping-around jeans, the kind of jeans you've owned for ten years and can wear to paint a room or clean a barn. They're ripped, stained, and crazy comfy. You wear them out when you're feeling bohemian. You wear them around the house, uh, everyday.

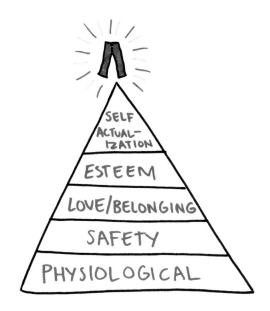

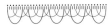
A particularly clumsy friend of mine was telling me that every season, like clockwork, she buys a pristine new pair of jeans, then falls in the street and rips the knees. She was dismayed by all the perfectly good jeans she'd been forced to toss into the cutoffs pile. "Why give up on them?" I asked. "The universe obviously wants you to bring back grunge." I convinced her to try out her ripped jeans with cute little cardigans, delicate necklaces, and basic black flats. She obliged, and guess who's rocking a new signature look?

Third Row (Love, Belonging): One pair of jeans that you secretly love but society deems shameful. For me, it's my pair of light denim overalls. For you, it may be a pair of tie-dyed cutoffs. You own these because they make you happy, and they're handy for testing the love and commitment of significant others. ("Would you still love me if I wore my overalls to the store with you today? Because I'm going to.")

Fourth Row (Esteem): This is the too-small pair of jeans that every woman keeps in the back of her closet, just in case she loses twenty pounds by accident. Try to limit yourself to just one (maaaayyybe two) of these, and keep them well hidden.

Fifth Row (Self-Actualization): The one pair of jeans that feel like they were made for you. Whenever you put them on, you want to tell the world "I just self-actualized in my pants!" even though it sounds dirty and inappropriate. If you haven't found your self-actualization jeans yet, don't worry. There's a pair out there for each of us.

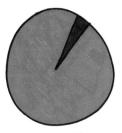

CORRECT

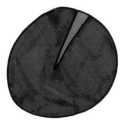

INCORRECT

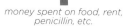

money spent on food, rent, penicillin, etc.

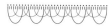

money spent on jeans

HOW MUCH TO SPEND

Over the past ten years, we've seen a shocking rise in the prices of jeans and water, two natural resources that used to be almost free. It didn't take long for the world to adjust to paying exorbitant sums of money for these items, nor to seamlessly integrate vocabulary like "premium denim" and "macrobiotic artesian water" into everyday conversation.

There was a time in my life, we'll call it my freshman year of college, when I spent approximately 95 percent of my monthly income on premium designer jeans and glass bottles of Italian water. I told myself that these thin pieces of cotton and inconveniently heavy canisters were wise investments, comparable to mutual funds. But here's the thing: I was being a dumbass. By the end of my glamorous year of Japanese denim and Italian water, my relationship with my credit card company had deteriorated almost as severely as my relationship with my LSD-popping roommate.

STYLE LESSON #3:

Premium jeans are quite wonderful, but they're not more wonderful than food, shelter, and a good credit rating.

I hate to sound like a credit counselor, but the number one consideration when deciding whether or not to splurge on expensive jeans is, can you afford to splurge? If you can, then go for it and don't look back. But if those jeans are going to plunge you into bankruptcy, either get another job and save up or consider one of the alternatives listed below.

Alternatives to Spending $300 on Jeans and Going Bankrupt

➤ **GO TO THE STORE,** figure out your size in your favorite designer jeans style, and then look for the same exact pair at discount stores and auction Web sites. I own quite a few pairs of premium denim that I scored for $60 or less because I knew which ones worked for me and jumped on some good deals.

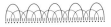

- ➤ **BUY A CHEAPER PAIR OF JEANS** and get crafty to make them special—add sequins on the pockets, spatter them with bleach, or dip-dye them in indigo. Seriously, put a little work into your jeans, and I swear you'll love them way more than any normal, boring, and expensive pair.

- ➤ **YOU COULD TRY TO SPLIT THE COST OF A PAIR OF PREMIUM JEANS** with your friends and hope for a *Sisterhood of the Traveling Pants*–type miracle, but I can't personally vouch for this method.

Now, say you're in a different boat and you can afford some spendy denim, but you're still not sure whether to fork over a couple hundred bucks or snag a pair of $5 sale bin stretch denim jeans from Sears (FYI—I've found some really good stuff in that sale bin). The best argument for shelling out the cheddar for premium jeans is that if you find a great pair, you're sure to wear them all the time. While ultratrendy, detailed, or fancy denim is usually the most costly, it doesn't make sense to spend a ton on

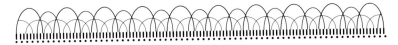

WHAT ABOUT COLORED JEANS?

I am a huge fan of brightly colored jeans. Let me tell you a little story to explain why. Once upon a time, I found a pair of neon yellow jeans languishing on a clearance rack. I picked them up, intending to mock them, only to find that they were my size and only $11. So I bought them instead.

The first time I wore them out of the house (it took me six months to work up the courage), I took a wrong turn on my walk home from the coffee shop. Within minutes, I found myself lugging my completely impractical bedazzled laptop bag and an overstuffed purse as I edged along the shoulder of a major thoroughfare in the dark, balancing between speeding traffic and a drainage ditch. As I approached a blind curve, I prepared to hurl myself into the abyss to avoid certain death; but then, the beams from the oncoming headlights caught my jeans, and suddenly my legs were glowing brighter than any safety vest. I was visible, invincible! That yellow denim lit my way home: oh yes, those colored jeans saved my life.

SHOULD I BRING A FRIEND SHOPPING WITH ME?

If you want the moral support, then absolutely, but I personally prefer to go it alone. That way, I feel freer to try on risky styles without judgment, and I can take my time deciding what I really like.

I TEND TO HAVE PROBLEMS WITH MUFFIN TOP— ANY SUGGESTIONS?

Ah, the muffin top. While the banana nut variety is delicious, the belly-bubbling-over-a-too-tight-waistband kind is extremely unappealing. Two strategies exist to combat this evil phenomenon: buy jeans with a bigger waist size than you're used to or, even better, go for a higher rise. Super-low-rise jeans can give even the most un-muffiny woman a fierce case of muffin top.

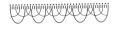

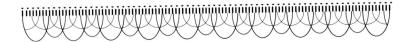

a pair of jeans you'll wear a couple of times a month. On the other hand, a great-fitting pair of versatile, everyday jeans from the bottom row of Maslow's Hierarchy is probably worth the money (basic shopping equation to remember: divide the price by the number of times you'll wear the item, and soon those pants are cutting you a check!). Higher costs often mean a higher level of quality, and for a wardrobe staple like a great pair of jeans, sometimes the shocking price tag makes sense. Sometimes.

GO FORTH AND CONQUER

Jeans shopping is no walk in the park (unless you go jeans shopping at an outdoor park sale, I suppose), but with a bit of planning and denim knowledge, you can alleviate much of the trauma. Study Maslow's Hierarchy and your handy Denim Field Guide, and take comfort in the fact that no matter our differences, women around the world are confused by terms like "curvy super low distressed button straight boot leg" and totally understand what it's like to be unable to fit an ankle into a completely unrealistic thigh-opening. So go forth and scour the racks for denim. Take a few pulls off your flask, then set it aside and try on more jeans than you ever thought you would—than you ever thought you'd need to. Try on skinny jeans and baggy jeans and dark jeans and light jeans. Slip on $5 sale bin jeans and $400 diamond-encrusted jeans. Power through the bad pairs and revel in the good. Trust me, you'll find denim self-actualization after all.

TWO

What to Wear on Top:

CHOOSING THE BEST SHIRTS, BLOUSES, BLAZERS, AND SWEATERS

TOPS ARE AN INTEGRAL PART OF EVERY WOMAN'S WARDROBE. They sort of have to be, unless you favor walking around in just a bra and a down jacket (if you actually do favor that, feel free to skip ahead to the lingerie and outerwear chapters). Having a good understanding of your separates and how to layer them is extremely helpful in both flattering your figure and carving out your personal style. Read on for lessons on responsible layering, overrated classics, underrated must-haves, and choosing the perfect ironic T-shirt.

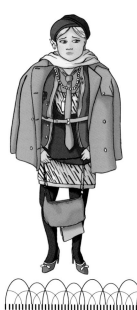

One of the most important fashion lessons a modern day woman can learn is how to layer shirts and tops in a fashionable, flattering way. Layering can be a fun technique to add interest to your outfits, but people often take the concept too far. I recently saw a fashion magazine feature titled "Spring Layering," but it was more like a snuff film in which the model is slowly strangled to death by shirts and sweaters and vests and coats. By the end, the poor model was wearing a tank top, a T-shirt, two sweaters, a vest, a skirt, a dress, two coats, and a pile of tangled necklaces; her smile was as strained as you'd expect from someone whose ribcage was slowly collapsing under four hundred pounds of cashmere. I could barely stand to look.

CHEZ DE SHIRT MENU

APPETIZERS
Tank top (choice of color
and fabric)
Camisole (with lace detail)
Camisole (no lace)
Vest

MAIN COURSES
Summer Selections
Cotton crewneck T-shirt
(served plain or with a
side of irony)
V-neck T-shirt
Button-up blouse
Cotton or silk tunic
Peasant blouse
Light cardigan

Linen blazer
Hoodie
Shrug

Winter Selections
Long-sleeved T-shirt
Button-up flannel (Seattle and
Portland locations only)
Tunic sweater
Turtleneck
Cardigan (served with
matching shell on request; also
ask about grandpa and
boyfriend varieties)
Hoodie
Blazer
Button-up oxford

SIDE DISHES
Stripe, polka-dot, or floral
patterns (à la carte)
Argyle print (served with
sweaters only)
Decorative buttons
Sequins
Elbow patches
Cable knit, tweed, or ribbed
textures (à la carte)
Ruffles or bows (choose one)

DESSERTS
Cashmere sweater
(market price)
Chunky-knit sweater
Sweater coat

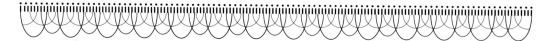

Layering different tops is a great way to spice up your look, but remember to prioritize lung function.

Spend a Sunday in your closet experimenting with different combinations of shirts, blouses, and sweaters, and I guarantee you'll be surprised by which pieces work really well together (a sequined shrug over a tuxedo shirt over a pink camisole? OK then!). And don't forget about the role of accessories in the layering process. One of my favorite clothing combinations is a polka-dot silk button-up blouse over a long tank top

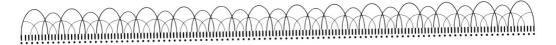

STYLISH, DELICIOUS COMBOS

Here are some layering recipes using items from the Chez de Shirt menu that are guaranteed to look good and allow you to breathe:

Vintage silk shirt
with bow at the neck
Slim-fitting black vest
Black blazer
Total: Professional plus

Cream lace camisole
Brown long-sleeved
cotton T-shirt
Blue cashmere cardigan
Total: Weekend getaway chic

Long hot-pink tank top
Shorter black tank top
Gray boyfriend sweater
Total: Movie-ready

Floral blouse with ruffles
Bright red sweater
Thin black belt
Total: Office adorable

Sequined racerback tank top
Black cardigan
Cropped white blazer
Total: Night-out nice

Lace camisole
Argyle cardigan
Total: Sexy nerdy

Silk T-shirt
Crisp white button-up oxford
Orange cashmere scarf
Total: Artistic eye

Red turtleneck
Black tank top
Total: Simple mod

Lace camisole
Blue and white striped
long-sleeved shirt
Oatmeal-colored chunky-
knit sweater
Total: Cozy Parisian

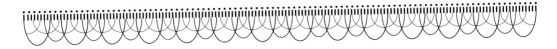

with a cardigan, all of which looks fairly insane until I throw on a pile of gold necklaces. Scarves have a similar effect. Often, it's the accessories that complete the look and bring it all together.

T-SHIRTS

Is there anything more iconic and all-American than the plain white T-shirt? Well, besides apple pie and baseball and shockingly bad romantic comedies? T-shirts are a part of our country's history (the founding fathers actually signed the Declaration of Independence while wearing matching tees—so adorable!), and they're a huge part of most of our wardrobes. A T-shirt most commonly has short sleeves and a crewneck and is made of cotton, although there are probably a million variations, made out of everything from satin to polyester to cashmere, with V-necks, scoop necks, or boatnecks. As a general rule, the further your T-shirt strays from the original formula of cotton crewneck, the more formal it is and the more places you can wear it. For example, a scoop neck satin "T-shirt" can be worn to the store, to work, or with a full ball skirt to the opera. For the purposes of this section, however, let's just focus on the classic crewneck cotton variety.

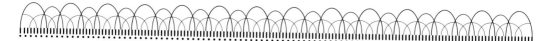

SPECIAL LAYERING MENU
(FOR SOME EXTRA IDEAS)

Pinstripe vest
Graphic tee
Banded collar blouse
Vintage lace bed jacket
Wrap shirt
Belted sweater

Cap sleeve shirt
Corset
Shawl
Wrap
Faux fur stole
Mini dress worn as top

Halter top
Off-the-shoulder top
Kimono sleeve top
Strapless top
(try it as an outer layer!)

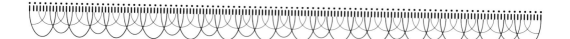

Graphic and Message T-Shirts

Graphic tees can be the coolest part of your wardrobe, or they can be supremely tacky. Acceptable graphic T-shirt subcategories include concert T-shirts (I wear my Spice Girls reunion tour T-shirt all the time), retro shirts, vintage political tees (anything vintage, for that matter), and those with funky bar logos or simple screen-printed designs. On the other hand, message T-shirts are usually pretty dire, especially those featuring stupid jokes ("Will Work For Beer!"). Also bad: Any shirt that includes the word "Hottie," the Playboy logo, or a tourist badge of pride ("Acapulco '03!").

And then there are the shirts that are so bad they're good: the yellow unicorn tee from the '80s, the well-worn "Virginia Is For Lovers" tee, or maybe even that "Acapulco '03!" monstrosity. Obviously, you must be vigilant about tops in this category. The current hipster culture dictates a very fine line between ironically cool and catastrophically stupid, so the ironic T-shirt is risky business indeed (note: a *Risky Business* T-shirt would probably be ironically cool). Not sure which side of the line your T-shirt falls on? Take the quiz on page 21 to find out.

NECKLINE LINEUP

The single most important feature of a top is the neckline. Sure, the color is notable, and the cut can mean the difference between looking like a sleek, modern woman or a mini-fridge with human legs, but the neckline frames your face, affects how the shirt hangs, and determines what parts of you are accentuated.

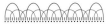

PLACES IT'S OK TO WEAR A T-SHIRT

House

School

Grocery store

Sporting events (playing or watching)

Gym

Beach

Casual dates

T-shirt Appreciation Club

Depending on your work environment, T-shirts may be acceptable, but stick to plain ones, make sure you wear them over or under something, keep the colors bright and crisp, and for the love of God, no stains

PLACES IT'S NOT OK TO WEAR A T-SHIRT

Weddings or funerals

Job interviews

Dinner parties

Bars in Mexico during spring break (unless you're into the whole wet T-shirt contest thing . . . then by all means)

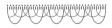

Once you find a neckline that suits your body, you'll feel enthused and confident and may want to make it your signature look. For example, I wear V-necks as regularly as an Italian mob boss.

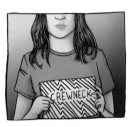

Crewneck

Notorious for: Making busty women appear even bustier

Vindicated for: Being a clean, classic look that never goes out of style

Known associates: T-shirts, sweaters, shells

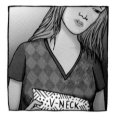

V-neck

Notorious for: Being worn by Italian mob bosses

Vindicated for: Being the busty girl's flattering alternative to crewnecks, visually elongating short necks

Known associates: T-shirts, sweaters, tank tops, tunics, Mafiosi

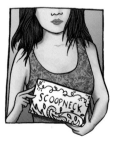

Scoop neck

Notorious for: Showing unexpected amounts of cleavage

Vindicated for: Showing unexpected amounts of cleavage

Known associates: T-shirts, sweaters, tank tops

The T-Shirt Test: Ironic or Just Lame?

Answer the following questions about your T-shirt, tallying your score
for all Yes answers (unless otherwise noted) as you go along:

1: **Does the shirt feature a communist
icon? (+50 points)**

➤ If yes, was it produced in a sweatshop
and sold at a big-box store
(such as Wal-Mart)? (–550 points)

2: **How many other people currently
own this shirt?**

➤ Less than 50 (shirt is vintage)?
(+100 points)
➤ Between 50 and 50,000 (shirt
promotes an obscure band)?
(+50 points)
➤ Over 50,000 (shirt is sold at the mall)?
(–100 points)

3: **Does the imagery/message on the
shirt reflect your personal tastes
or beliefs? (For example, if you own
a "Dungeons and Dragons Club"
T-shirt, are you actually a member of
the Dungeons and Dragons Club?)**

➤ Yes (–500 points)
➤ No (+500 points)

4: **Please choose the adjective set
that most accurately describes the
size of your shirt:**

➤ Oversized, baggy (–100 points)
➤ Slim-fitting, body-conscious
(+100 points; add an additional
500 bonus points if shirt is tight
enough to show your heartbeat)

5: **Does the shirt show wear
and tear?**

➤ Yes (+50 points; double
this if the shirt also features
a communist icon)
➤ No (–100 points)

6: **How much did the shirt cost?**

➤ Less than $10 (+50 points)
➤ More than $10 (–50 points)
➤ Nothing, you found it in a dumpster
(+1,000 points)

Now, add up your score. If the number
is positive, congratulations! Your shirt is
ironic and cool (the higher your number,
the cooler the tee). If your shirt scored
a negative, I'm sorry, but it's my responsibility to tell you that it's probably lame.

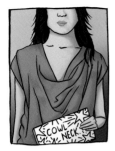

Cowl neck

Notorious for: Sometimes looking kind of strange

Vindicated for: Adding interest to plain shirts, bringing attention up to the neck and face

Known associates: Tank tops, sweaters, tunics

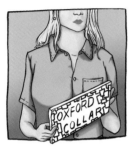

Oxford collar

Notorious for: Making short necks look stumpier, not living up to the hype

Vindicated for: Looking really crisp and credible at the office

Known associates: Cotton, poplin, polyester

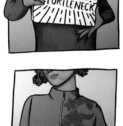

Turtleneck

Notorious for: Being the go-to shirt choice of kindergarteners

Vindicated for: Keeping your neck warm

Known associates: Ribbed cotton, sweaters

Mockneck

Notorious for: Impersonating the turtleneck, albeit unconvincingly

Vindicated for: Hmm . . . can't think of anything

Known associates: My friend Rachel once received a green velour mockneck tank top as a gift; ten years later, we're still talking about how horrifically ugly it was

Halter

Notorious for: Refusing to work with bras

Vindicated for: Accentuating lovely necks and shoulders

Known associates: Cotton, silk, swimsuits

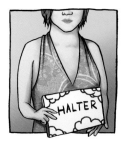

Polo collar

Notorious for: Being popped up by frat guys

Vindicated for: Making retail store employees easy to spot

Known associates: Cotton-poly blend, board shorts, Pabst Blue Ribbon

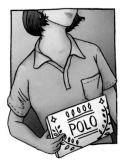

FIVE TOPS THAT LOOK GOOD ON EVERYONE

➤ **THE T-SHIRT**
As I noted above, this simple shirt can't be worn everywhere, but it can be worn by everyone. Different necklines flatter different figures: make sure to find your ideal T-shirt before you die.

➤ **THE WRAP SHIRT**
Put on a wrap shirt, especially a sheer cashmere wrap shirt, and you'll feel like a ballerina. This is the shirt of lost childhood dreams.

➤ **THE VEST**
From cropped tweed varieties to slouchy knit options, vests are cute, versatile, and super flattering.

➤ **THE V-NECK SWEATER**
A V-neck sweater in a great color will never do you wrong. Try a deep V-neck to layer over pretty camisoles.

➤ **THE BLACK CARDIGAN**
I sing the praises of the black cardigan with great passion later in the chapter, so here I'll just say, if you don't have a black cardigan yet, go buy one. Seriously, right now. Put the book down. Go!

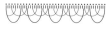
I believe the white button-up shirt is perhaps the most overrated, overhyped piece of clothing in history. I know, I know, every credible fashion and news source insists that the white oxford shirt is a MUST-HAVE that makes everyone look like a slim, sexy secretary. Unfortunately, my experiences with white button-up shirts usually go more like this:

I wake up in the morning and need to get ready for work. I have nothing to wear, and I get upset about this. I spy a wadded-up white oxford shirt jammed into the back of my closet. "I can't imagine why this was obviously shoved back here in a rage," I think, and with visions of confident, sexy career woman dancing through my head, I un-wad the shirt and

AND THREE TOPS
THAT LOOK GOOD ON NO ONE

➤ THE BOXY SILK SHIRT

Boxy shapes are unflattering. Silk magnifies unflattering features. No good can come of this combo.

➤ THE SKINTIGHT SPANDEX ANYTHING

Save the skintight spandex for cross-country cycling trips. And even then, give it some thought.

➤ THE PONCHO

These vast swaths of fabric make anyone look like a triangular mass with stumpy arms. However, I must admit that along with overalls, ponchos are one of my secret fashion guilty pleasures. Don't judge.

STYLE LESSON #6:

If oxford shirts actually work for you, then you should totally wear them every day; if not, don't force it. A slim-fitting cardigan or a silk blouse can easily create the same level of sexy professionalism without the emotional trauma.

SWEATERS

Rarely am I *not* wearing a sweater. In winter, you'll find me in chunky-knit wrap sweaters, thick cardigans, grandpa sweaters (see sidebar on page 26), and cozy cashmere. In the warmer months, I still throw on a light cotton cardigan pretty much every day and keep sweater coats close at hand for chilly summer nights. If a sweater asked for my hand in marriage, I would probably say yes.

Some General Tips for Shopping for Sweaters

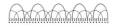

➤ **IT'S A RARE SITUATION** where you actually need to buy a full-priced sweater. Stores are crazy, so they put out their fall and winter selections during the heat of summer. Wait until you're actually a little chilly to shop for sweaters, and you'll find the same huge selection on sale.

➤ **IF YOU'D LIKE TO SAVE EVEN MORE MONEY,** look for sweaters at thrift stores. Some of my favorite grandpa cardigans were no doubt previously owned by grandpas, and you can't beat good quality cashmere thrifted for under $10.

➤ **INVEST IN BASIC SWEATERS** you'll wear all the time. In my college days, I spent hundreds of dollars on about fifteen inexpensive black cardigans (my trademark), when I could have invested in one quality piece and still had it to this day. Alas, the foolish things we do in our early twenties.

➤ **BELTED SWEATERS ARE APPEALING** and look fantastic on some people, but beware: the bulky fabric plus the belt can make you look about a foot wider around the middle.

➤ **UNLESS YOU ARE THE QUEEN OF ENGLAND,** matching sweater sets should be avoided.

Speaking of Cardigans . . .

I'm a huge fan of the cardigan sweater. Cardigans literally look good on everyone (play with different lengths, colors, and necklines to find your perfect combo) and can add some wonderful variety to your wardrobe. Throw a colorful cardigan over the most boring outfit ever and trust me, you'll look instantly fresh and fabulous. Conversely, throw a black cardigan over pretty much anything—a ribbed white tank, a summer dress, a fishnet bodysuit—and you'll look instantly put together and very nearly work appropriate.

The fact that cardigans look good over anything doesn't mean you should wear them over just anything. I used to use my collection of cute, flattering cardigans as a sort of sartorial glue to hold together an otherwise problematic and unedited wardrobe. My cardigans were like that one really fun, easy-to-get-along-with friend that you drag to lame parties because you know she'll make them fun. Of course, after a while you begin to wonder, why am I going to these bad parties in the first place? In my case, the bad party was a collection of tank tops and T-shirts that

put it on. As I skip out the door to work, I feel good; I feel like I'm wearing what a hot young professional is supposed to wear. Then, at some point during the day, I catch a glimpse of myself in a mirror, and my oxford shirt fantasies come crashing down around me: the shirt is wrinkled, the buttons are gaping, I've dribbled bits of my lunch onto the white fabric, and the stiff collar is doing nothing for my already short neck. I look rumpled and at least double my age. This is the one thing every woman should have in her wardrobe?

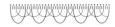

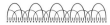

WHAT THE HELL IS A GRANDPA SWEATER?

A grandpa sweater (also known as an "old man sweater") is, as you might have guessed, a sweater that looks like something a grandpa would wear. If you've never seen your grandpa wear a sweater, picture Mr. Rogers and his cardigan collection. The most common incarnation of the grandpa sweater is the oversized cardigan. While this style of sweater looks sort of awkward and quaint when worn by an actual grandpa, when adopted by a young woman and thrown over a flouncy dress or a tank top and jeans, it is suddenly a sexy, stylish statement piece. Double points if you actually got your grandpa sweater from your grandpa.

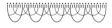

didn't really fit me and that I would never wear on their own. My solution? Throw on a cardigan! But whenever I would throw one on over, say, a stained, too-tight pink tank top, extraordinary circumstances would inevitably force me to take off the cardigan, and then it was just me and my stained, too-tight pink tank top.

STYLE LESSON #7:

Whatever you wear under your cardigan, make sure it fits well and looks just as good on its own. What if you walk by the scene of a biking accident and the first responders cry out, "We need a tourniquet! Ma'am, give us your sweater!"? Do you want to be the woman who runs the other way, shouting, "I'm so sorry, but I'd rather not show the world this marinara stain!"?

BLAZERS

My first experience with a blazer took place in my teens and involved a boxy, mustard green corduroy version I found on a clearance rack. It was one of those pieces of clothing that triggers a daily cycle of denial—I would put it on almost every morning thinking it would look great, and of course it looked just as horrible as it had the day before; naturally, I would go through the same process again the next day.

I took this blazer with me when I moved into the dorm my freshman year of college. Sure, I tried it on one more time before I packed it, and it looked awful, but I decided my new college self was definitely the kind of person who wore blazers, especially those of the boxy, mustard green corduroy variety.

One day, while getting ready for a dining hall dinner, I spotted the wretched thing in the drawer beneath my bed and decided it was time for its university debut. I was just a few feet out the door when I caught a glimpse of myself in a window and stopped. I gaped at what I assumed was my reflection, although it might as well have been a frumpy farm-hand staring at me in disgust from the other side of the glass. The view was so unflattering I stripped off the blazer right there in the hall and flagged down a Scandinavian exchange student who happened to be walking by. "Hey," I said flatly, "do you want this?"

"Sure," she said, and skipped away singing the praises of the generous American spirit.

I didn't wear a blazer again until a few years later, when I discovered a basic black one I couldn't resist trying on. Completely the opposite of the mustard corduroy incarnation, my find was so flattering that I didn't take it off for three months. I layered it with T-shirts, ribbed tank tops, silk mini dresses, and sweaters. I rolled up the sleeves and threw it on over sheer T-shirts and denim cutoffs in the summer and thick tights, printed skirts, and cashmere turtlenecks in the winter. I wore it with men's ties and women's scarves and dangly earrings and yellow curry (I'm a messy eater).

STYLE LESSON #8:

A black blazer, like a black cardigan and a black peacoat, is an absolute, no-question, non-negotiable must-have.

If you already own one, you're probably familiar with its magical powers of figure flattery and its ability to morph back and forth effortlessly between trendy and professional. However, if you don't have one, you should definitely get yourself to the mall. Here's what to look for:

Buttons

Start with the single-breasted style—it's most flattering and versatile. Go for five buttons at the most and two at the fewest (one can be OK, but if the fit is even a little snug, that button is going to look miiiiiiigggghty strained). Most women, no matter their chest size, look good in a three-button blazer with a nipped-in waist, while very few women look good in a twenty-button blazer.

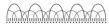

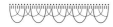
Shoulders

Look for a blazer that fits comfortably in the shoulders. You should be able to cross your arms in front of you without causing a catastrophic seam explosion in the back. Shoulders with a bit of a stiff shape can be really flattering, but steer clear of shoulder pads.

Shape

Ladies who are straight up and down or wider in the middle should regard the fitted blazer as a wondrous blessing. Many blazers are structured in hourglass shapes that can fool the world into thinking you are too. Most everyone should avoid boxy styles, but have fun experimenting with cropped blazers, longer styles, and looser shapes.

COLOR

Shirts, sweaters, and blazers are your opportunity to bring color close to your face and really brighten your whole appearance, so it's worthwhile to know what colors work best for you. A good place to start when figuring out your optimum shirt hues is your hair color. See the following illustration for some of the best color options for you:

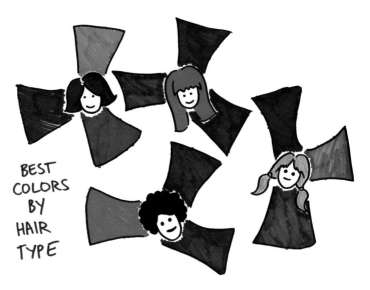

BEST COLORS BY HAIR TYPE

TOP IT OFF

Sure, you can layer a tank top under a vest under a cardigan under a blazer under a scarf and look fabulous, but sometimes this approach is neither necessary nor desirable. A silk tunic in a gorgeous color, a bejeweled sweater, a polka-dot button-up shirt, a ruffle-necked blouse—many tops are so lovely and eye-catching on their own that it's best to simply let them steal the show.

If layering isn't your thing, or if you want to change up your usually layered look for a night out, try a feminine blouse with special details like sequins, beadwork, textured fabric, embroidery, or a satin sash. Play around with belted shapes, longer tops, and embellished necklines. Don't wear anything you don't feel comfortable in, of course, but remember that sometimes, your perfect shirt is hanging on a rack just outside your comfort zone. And it's probably on sale.

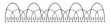

4. Clue:
A little flash for a girls' night out, wear this combo and you're sure to stand out.

Answer:
Blazer + Sequined tank top

5. Clue:
This one is simple and fashionable too; give it a try—you'll be glad if you do!

Answer:
Blazer + Simple tank top or T-shirt

6. Clue:
Hop in a time machine and here's what you'll see: this popular style at Prom '83.

Answer:
Blazer + Ruffled tuxedo shirt

7. Clue:
This style is a classic and often seen; go anywhere "Business Casual" and you'll know what I mean.

Answer:
Blazer + Classic oxford shirt

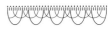

THREE

Below the Belt:

YOUR GUIDE TO SKIRTS, PANTS, AND SHORTS

I AM AN APPLE, OR A WATERMELON, SOMETIMES. My friend Rachel is a pear. My friend Jennifer is celery.

If a man were to read those sentences, he would probably assume my friends and I were starting a second-rate pop music group called The Produce Girls, and while that would be sort of amazing (just call me Apple Spice), he would be mistaken. If a woman were to read those sentences, she would simply nod in understanding and possibly add, "I'm a pear, too."

It seems as long as fashion advice has existed, fashion advisors have been grouping women into body type categories and addressing each group as the fruit or vegetable it most resembles. Someone with a round stomach (like me, for example) is often called an apple. Women with larger hips and thighs are referred to as pears. And so it goes.

I've always found this practice pretty annoying, not to mention a little insulting. (In the seventh grade, a friend of mine burst out crying at a slumber party because *Vogue* deemed her a cinnamon stick.) When we're talking about skirts and pants, it does make sense to discuss the best options in terms of specific body types, but I don't think it's necessary to assign every woman a role in a seasonal fruit salad.

STYLE LESSON #9:

Understand your shape in order to
dress your best, but always remember:
you are much more
than a pear.

BEST BOTTOMS FOR YOUR BODY

If your hips and thighs are significantly
larger than your waist, you are
a ~~pear~~ Beautiful Grecian Goddess

THE GOOD:

➤ **Pants labeled "curvy"** "Curvy" pants are made for you. This label usually means some extra room in the hips and thighs and a tapered waist, which prevents that dreaded gaping waistband in the back.

➤ **Flared legs** Whether a simple boot cut or a full-on flare, this shape looks fantastic on you.

- **Wide-leg trousers** This style of pants is extremely flattering and fashionable. Pair these voluminous bottoms with a body-skimming shirt, structured blazer, or fitted cardigan for a modern silhouette.

- **Skinny pants** Try using tight pants as a base layer. Get yourself a pair of skinny black pants, for example, and pair them with tunics or mini dresses that flow over your hips and thighs. This look is very pretty and always in style. Try tops in eye-catching colors like peacock blue and gorgeous fabrics like satin.

- **Knee-length shorts** Try a pair of shorts that hit just above the knees (or just below if you're not a fan of your knees) for summer, or create your own by cutting off a pair of jeans.

- **Magical universally flattering skirt** (see sidebar)

- **Peasant skirts** These hippie-chic, flowy bottoms are perfect for weekend outings and hot summer days. They're just as airy and cool as miniskirts but don't reveal nearly as much skin. Try a colorful peasant skirt with a black ribbed tank top and simple sandals.

THE BAD:

- **Khaki capri pants**
- **Super-low-rise pants**
- **Cargo shorts**

THE AWESOME EXTRAS:

- **Boots** A pair of boots is a stylish addition to any outfit. This is especially true for Beautiful Grecian Goddesses, because boots—the more rugged the better—act as an anchor for large hips. Dainty shoes, like kitten-heeled sandals, can make legs seem larger, but boots are a way to even things out. Wear your big black boots with dark tights and a knee-length dress for optimal figure flattery and style.

- **Belts** A belt around your natural waist creates a focal point above your hips and defines a slim torso. Wrap a skinny red belt (or a couple!) around a black cardigan, throw on a flared skirt and some boots, and thank me in the morning.

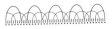

THE SKIRT THAT REALLY, TRULY, SWEAR-ON-MY-MOTHER'S-LIFE LOOKS GOOD ON EVERYONE (INCLUDING MY MOTHER)

Knee-length, slightly A-line skirts are one of those rare fashion creations that don't just look passable on every body type—they make every body type look better. This style of skirt grazes over large hips, adds curves to svelte figures, complements hourglass shapes, and flares out attractively from bigger bellies. To say that this skirt might possess magical powers would be a gross underestimation of its abilities. This skirt definitely possesses magical powers.

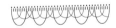

If your waist is larger than your hips, you are an ~~apple~~ Stellar Soft Siren

THE GOOD:

➤ **Pants with a medium rise** Repeat after me, sweet siren: low-rise pants are not a friend. In fact, they are sworn enemies who conspire to make you look bloated. Also, as I mentioned in the jeans chapter, if you don't tuck in your shirt, high-waisted pants are just a girdle. And we sirens love us a good girdle.

➤ **Boot cut and straight leg pants** Trousers with a bit of a flare or a crisp, straight leg are extremely flattering. Bonus points for pinstripes or vertical seams.

➤ **Magical universally flattering skirt** (see sidebar on page 33)

➤ **Midthigh length shorts** In the summertime, choose the shortest shorts you feel comfortable in—usually a good fashion rule of thumb—to elongate your legs and draw attention down and away from your belly.

➤ **Miniskirts** Many women who carry their weight in their stomachs are blessed with beautiful, shapely legs that deserve to be shown off, so try shorter skirts in slightly flared shapes for weekends or date nights.

THE BAD:

➤ **Belts** (see Style Lesson #31)

➤ **Wide-leg trousers**

➤ **Pencil skirts**

THE AWESOME EXTRAS:

➤ **Wide waistbands** Wide waistbands hold in your belly and create a smoother base for your tops. What's not to love?

➤ **Detailed hems** Skirts with fun details like ruffles, bows, or lace at the hem draw attention down toward your fabulous gams and add general interest to your outfit.

If your torso and hips are very straight up and down, you are a ~~celery stick~~ Lovely Lithe Lady

THE GOOD:

➤ **Low-rise pants** Low-rise pants widen the hips visually, which is why they're not the best option for large-hipped ladies but are an excellent choice for you. Add a statement-making belt for extra oomph.

➤ **Boot cut pants** Pants with a slight flare create a subtly curvy leg line without looking contrived.

➤ **Menswear-inspired pants** Roomier trousers add some bulk to smaller hips and always look fashion forward. For work, try a pair of loose tweed pants slung low on your hips with a slim-fitting silk blouse in a pretty color; for a fun weekend look, experiment with pleated pants rolled at the hems with a simple tank top.

➤ **Short shorts** If you'd like to draw attention to lean legs, sport the shortest shorts you feel comfortable in. Add a flowy tunic top for a modern shape.

➤ **Capri pants** Capris are a tricky style for most body types, but lucky Lovely Lithe Ladies can usually pull them off looking more like Audrey Hepburn than a harried soccer mom.

➤ **Magical universally flattering skirt** (see sidebar on page 33)

➤ **Swingy skirts** There are so many fun skirts with fullness and movement to choose from—keep an eye out for features like shiny fabrics, multiple layers, interesting hemlines, ruffles, or all of the above!

THE BAD:

➤ **Super–flared pants**

➤ **Boxy skirts**

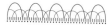

**HOW TO FIND
THE BEST
(AND WORST) PANTS
LENGTH FOR YOU!**

You will need:

**One pair of old
jeans or slacks**

Scissors

A mirror

Step 1:
*Lay old pants on the
floor and use scissors to
cut off about two inches
of fabric at the hem.*

Step 2:
Put pants on.

Step 3:
*Look in mirror. Do you
look like a hobbit? If yes,
repeat steps 1–3 until
you find the best
length for you.*

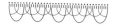

THE AWESOME EXTRAS:

➤ **Pant cuffs** A crisp cuff on a trouser leg gives more weight to the bottom of your silhouette and creates a really flattering shape.

➤ **Belts** When your figure is fairly straight, you can carve out a waist illusion with a belt—wrap one around wherever you'd like your waist to be, and ta-da!

If you have an hourglass figure, you are a ~~gourd~~ Marilyn Monroe

THE GOOD:

➤ **Pencil skirts** An hourglass shape looks undeniably amazing in a pencil skirt, so there's basically no excuse not to wear one.

➤ **High-waisted trousers** Play up your striking shape with the retro look of high-waisted, flare leg trousers, which draw attention to a small waist.

➤ **Pants labeled "curvy"** As I mentioned in the Grecian Goddess section, finding pants that fit big hips without gaping in the back can be tough. "Curvy" pants are usually constructed specifically for women blessed with curves.

➤ **Shorts that hit just above the knee** While retro styles obviously look great on you, steer clear of short shorts to avoid looking like you belong in a pinup calendar (unless that's the look you're going for).

➤ **Capri pants** Your balanced figure means that cropped pants have the potential to look great on you. Try slim slacks that hit a few inches above your ankles with a pair of cute flats and a black cardigan.

➤ **Magical universally flattering skirt** (see sidebar on page 33)

THE BAD:

➤ **Super-flared skirts**

➤ **Anything baggy**

THE AWESOME EXTRAS:

➤ **Fabulous hosiery** Add a pair of lace tights to your outfit and feel yourself *strut* down the hallway to the copy machine.

➤ **Belts** Show off your amazing waist with a spotlight-grabbing belt. Wear it through belt loops, over a sweater, slung over your hips, whatever—but do wear it!

THE CANKLE QUANDARY

As we discuss how to dress your bottom half, we cannot ignore the cankle quandary. Many women despair over their self-diagnosed "cankles" (a clever blend of "calves" and "ankles," for those lucky enough never to have heard the term), believing themselves to be doomed to a gloomy life of long pants because of their thick legs.

Now, before I offer my own tips, let me just say that I despise the default fashion advice that is dispensed to short and/or stocky-legged women: "High heels are a must! Always wear heels! Really, really high heels!"

STYLE LESSON #10:

Real women can't "just wear heels" all of the time, and even if we could, we wouldn't want to.

Now that that's out of the way, let's get to some realistic cankle-fighting options:

➤ **WEDGES.** Wedges are high heels' kinder, gentler, and equally flattering cousin. They are magical in their ability to give you some height (and therefore elongate the leg) while maintaining comfort. Even a small wedge will make your legs look longer and slimmer.

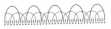

DRESSING ROOM DIARIES

Growing up, I had friends whose parents were very strict about the distinction between "school clothes" and "play clothes." These friends had two sections in their closets, and if I went to play with one of these friends after school, I had to wait around for them to carefully hang up their school clothes on the stiff hangers and retrieve an appropriate play outfit from the grimier section.

I was endlessly jealous of these friends as I sat there, watching them maintain two completely separate wardrobes. It seemed so exotic, so luxurious. My parents were more of the mind that all of our clothes would eventually be ruined (correct), so we might as well wear ruinable clothes to school. I proved Mom and Dad right every day by falling in mud puddles or offering to help clean up chocolate milk spills with my shirt.

continues »

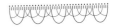

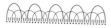

continued ▸

While the school clothes vs. play clothes divide seemed epic to me as a child, I didn't think much of it in adulthood until my friend Sarah mentioned a certain pair of school-only blue cords she'd had when she was a kid. She'd loved them so much, she would try to sneak them into her weekend outfits, but her mom would scold her and take them right back to the closet. Even into her twenties, Sarah dutifully and robotically came home from work and switched into ugly "play clothes" for evenings and weekends. But gradually, she started wearing her cool tweed trousers with a T-shirt and scarf for Sunday brunch, and her printed satin skirt with a tank top and heels for a night out. She absolutely loved her new sartorial freedom, and she realized that it doesn't make any sense to save your best clothes for work: life outside of work is where you really want to show your style.

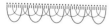

➤ **MAXI DRESSES.** I used to think that only models could pull off these easy, breezy, ankle-covering, floor-length dresses. Then one day, a short, normal-sized girl waltzed onto the bus wearing the cutest floor-length black jersey number, and my life was forever changed. She looked amazing, and for all I knew, her calves could have been the size of coffee cans. Pair with some stylish sandals and a few bracelets in the summer and you're good to go.

➤ **EYE-CATCHING TOPS.** Ah yes, the old bait and switch. Actually, come to think of it, I'm not sure what bait and switch means, but it seems right in this context. Wear a fabulous top with knee-length dark denim jeans, and I swear nobody will notice your legs (not in a bad way, anyway).

➤ **BOOTS.** Depending on the climate, of course, because dying of heat-stroke in an effort to conceal your cankles would be a very sad way to go. But generally speaking, boots are a wonderful choice for cankle concealment. Get a worn-in pair you can wear with dresses in the summer as a hip and flattering alternative to flats or sandals.

AVOID:

➤ **EXTRA DAINTY SHOES.** It's all about proportions. People with large heads do not look their best in wee little newsboy caps. Similarly, larger legs will not look their best in wee little shoes.

➤ **GLADIATOR SANDALS.** This difficult style of footwear has the power to make a supermodel look like Danny DeVito. Not. Good.

➤ **SKIRTS OR PANTS THAT HIT MIDCALF.** As a short person, I've found that this length is the most stumpifying. Whenever I try on something with a hemline in this danger zone, I frown at my suddenly even shorter legs in the mirror for a while, then realize that I can simply yank the hem up a few inches (or roll my pant legs down a few inches) to make the length super-flattering.

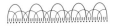

STYLE LESSON #11:

Wear your school pants to play and your play pants to school. You'll have more fun and make your mom nervous, and isn't that what life's all about?

IN A BLACK PANTS RUT?

It's inevitable that you will, at some point in your life, fall into a rut of wearing the same black pants (or gray trousers, or red pencil skirt . . .) every day. You get up every morning, look in your closet, lament your lack of anything to wear, and slip on those trusty standbys day after day. An easy remedy for this situation is a shopping spree, but if you'll allow me to speak on behalf of your closet space and credit card balance for a moment, I'd like to suggest an alternative strategy: take inventory first—shop second.

Taking inventory of your closet will help you remember all the pants and skirts that hang neglected in your closet, get rid of the ones you never wear, and give you a clear mission when you finally do go shopping. Set an afternoon aside, put on some music, and try to have some fun with this project.

Closet Inventory: Pants

Gather all of the pants you own and spread them out on your bed or the floor. I strongly advise you to do this when there is no chance of a man walking in on you, because if one does, he will take one look at the pile, stagger back dramatically, and then lecture you on how he has never owned more than three pairs of pants in his ENTIRE life and he isn't planning to buy another pair for at least a decade.

Divide the pants into three piles: pairs you wear all the time, pairs you wear sometimes, and pairs you never wear that you rescued from the dark depths of your closet.

For each pile, create a two-column list, describing each pair and why you love them, don't wear them often, or never wear them. For example, for pants you wear all the time, write down why you wear them so

THREE ALTERNATIVES TO PAYING A TAILOR TO HEM YOUR PANTS (IF YOU'RE AS CLUELESS ABOUT SEWING AS I AM)

Hack off the bottoms with scissors, roll up the hems a couple times to hide the uneven fraying, and voila— cuffed pants!

Ask an elderly relative to do it for you.

Put a piece of steak in the pocket. Throw the pants into a pack of wild dogs and hope the legs come out shorter.

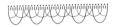

frequently—Are they really comfortable? Are they an integral part of your favorite outfit? Give your answers some thought, and be specific. See example below.

For the pants you wear all the time, answer the following questions:

➤ **Which features draw you** to these pants and keep you coming back?

➤ **Which body part do you like** your pants to accentuate?

➤ **Which body part do you like** your pants to de-emphasize?

➤ **What color pants** do you wear most often? Why?

➤ **Are you happy** with the pants you wear all the time? Would you like your go-to pants selection to be more varied or is it just right?

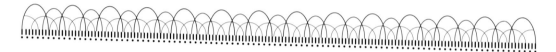

WEAR-ALL-THE-TIME PILE

Description

Black slim-leg slacks

Reason for Loving Them

Make my butt look amazing

When you're sorting through the Wear Sometimes and the Never Wear piles, focus on what is keeping each pair of pants out of the Wear-All-the-Time pile. If they're simply too formal or too memorable to wear all the time, that's fine; but usually these piles are stocked with old, stained, ill-fitting pants that you swore you'd take to the dry cleaners back in the day when "dry cleaners" meant "an old woman with a washboard by the river." Take a close look at each of these pants, and figure out what needs to be done. Do you need to rent a dump truck for a massive trip to the junkyard? Perhaps it's just a matter of moving some forgotten pants to the front of your closet. Or maybe you should have a few pairs properly tailored and give the rest to your unsuspecting niece ("Brown polyester bell bottoms?! Thanks, Aunt Winona!"). However you end up dealing with these piles, the key is to deal with them—the sooner the better.

Closet Inventory: Skirts

I think skirts, even more than pants, tend to get shoved into the backs of our closets and tragically forgotten. It's easy to keep pushing that teal satin skirt farther into the darkness, assuming it's just for parties and formal occasions, but then you neither see nor think of it when you're searching for a sassy bottom to pair with a white T-shirt and sandals in July.

As you did with pants, create three piles and three corresponding lists for your skirts. Divide once again into Wear-All-the-Time, Wear Sometimes, and Never Wear piles. When you're doing your skirt inventory, try to rethink your ideas of which skirts are work skirts, which are weekend skirts, which are fancy skirts, etc., because these pieces are almost always more versatile than they seem.

After completing the Wear-All-the-Time pile, answer the following questions:

➤ **What is it about these skirts** that makes you reach for them again and again? Interesting patterns? Cool shapes? Are they all the same length?

➤ **Are you bored** with your selection?

➤ **What type of skirt** would you like to wear but don't? Why not?

When all lists are complete, move your rarely worn and never worn skirts to the front of your closet, and spend a week trying to work them into your daily outfits. If you still don't like a skirt after a test wearing, it's probably not the skirt for you, but be open-minded, especially with your "formal" skirts—they can probably come out to see the light more often than you think.

With a thorough closet inventory, you could find enough previously forgotten bottoms in your closet to last you a decade. Of course, you still have my full permission to go shopping for more next week.

Common Problems and Suggested Solutions For the Pants and Skirts You Encounter During Your Closet Inventory

PROBLEM	SOLUTION
SLIGHTLY DIRTY	Take to the cleaners
SEVERELY STAINED	Take to the dump
MISSING A BUTTON	Replace button
MISSING A BUTTON, ZIPPER, AND TWO MAJOR SEAMS	Replace entire garment
A LITTLE TIGHT	Have them altered or give them away, but quick, before they zap your self-esteem
A LITTLE BIG	Keep 'em around for the day after . . . the buffet
REALLY TIGHT	Keep 'em around for the day after . . . food poisoning at the buffet
REALLY BIG	Have them altered or rock them as baggy menswear
A LITTLE UGLY	Pair with pretty tops for a trendy contrast
REALLY UGLY	Save for potential Halloween costume

FOUR

A Good Foundation Is Essential:

HOW BRAS, UNDERWEAR, NIGHTWEAR, AND HOSIERY CAN CHANGE YOUR LIFE

WHEN I WAS ABOUT TEN, I overheard my parents talking in hushed, serious tones about the fate of a seventeen-year-old neighbor girl who had driven her grandfather's tractor up a steep incline, flipped it, and become trapped underneath. While not seriously injured, she was wedged firmly between the colossal machine and the ground. As the paramedics heroically began to cut her out of her clothes to free her, they heard a scream: "This is a new bra! Get those scissors the hell away from me!" It took an hour of pleading and a promise that the paramedics would all chip in to buy her a new one for her to acquiesce. The bra was snipped, the tractor was lifted, and a style lesson was learned: *Never underestimate the importance of good undergarments.*

This story affected me profoundly and served as my guiding theme while writing this chapter. The things you wear under your clothes can make you look better and feel sexier. They're worth taking seriously. Even when trapped under a tractor.

LIFT AND SEPARATE: MY BRA STORY

Like all the women in the entire world (with the exception of those lucky tribal gals in Africa and Australia, I suppose), my first bra-buying experience ranked somewhere between Chinese water torture and eating hair.

Many writing manuals tell you to rhapsodize about your first love to find inspiration and good material, but I would like to propose that the women of the world tackle a subject much more interesting, emotionally intense, and worthy of documentation: their first bras.

Here's my entry:

My brassiered life began in the sixth grade. It was recess, and I was telling my friend Brittany all the reasons I didn't think I needed a bra yet, when it started raining. After a few minutes of rain and my anti-bra lecturing, Brittany interrupted me and pointed at my chest. I looked down to see that only my boobs were wet, and not much was left to the imagination beneath the damp spots on my thin, magenta JCPenney turtleneck. "Oh God," I whispered as I covered my chest and ran into the girls' bathroom. I knew that I had just become a woman. It was definitely a "this is the first day of the rest of your life" moment.

The next day I went to Mervyns with my mom to buy a bra. The salesclerk, a harsh German woman with a dangerously sharp-looking chest, took one look at me and declared, in a screech loud enough for the men in the tool section to hear, "We need to LIFT! And SEPARATE!"

I left with a gray jersey soft cup atrocity that looked more like a crudely constructed breast sling than a bra, and I've spent the rest of my life rewarding myself with expensive and impractical lingerie to make up for the experience.

I encourage you to write about your first bra-buying experience, and perhaps submit the story to a prestigious literary magazine.

You Gotta Get Fit

To paraphrase a line from *Fight Club*, the first rule of having boobs is: get a bra fitting. Something like 200 percent of women wear the wrong bra size. I think the official rule, handed down by ~~God~~ Oprah, is to get fitted once a year, or after any major weight gain or loss, but I'm such a passionate proponent of bra fittings that I get refitted pretty much any time I buy a new bra. Yes, sometimes the clerks are like, "Winona, seriously, your boobs are the same size they were yesterday," but I don't care. I'm on a quest for the perfect bra the way most people are on a quest for the meaning of life. In fact, if I was ever on a mountain-climbing expedition in Nepal and ran into a Buddhist wise man, I'd ask him if I should be wearing a demi or a full cup.

How Much to Spend

Throughout my childhood, my mom stressed the importance of a good bra to my three brothers and me. She would often line us up and have us repeat the phrase "A good foundation is essential," until we could say it back to her, verbatim. She would test my brothers at random intervals, summoning them from the backyard to ask, "No matter how poor you are or how many bills you have to pay, what is the one thing you will always buy for your wife?"

"A good bra!" my brothers would declare confidently, and then, with a nod of my mom's head, they were allowed to continue playing. I strongly suggest doing the same with your children, to impart good values and financial priorities.

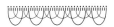

While it's not imperative to spend hundreds of dollars on a bra made by a skilled French craftsman named Pierre DeBrassiere, it's important that you don't skimp on quality.

Here's my advice: $30. If you go bra shopping and plan to spend about $30, you'll be able to enjoy fair-quality bras that cost $30, and more expensive bras marked down to $30. It's a good and reliable price point that has served me well for most of my bra-wearing life. Sometimes I accidentally buy $100 bras (those saleswomen are like ninjas and the lace is so pretty!), but hey, a good foundation is essential.

Your Burning Bra Questions, Answered

Can I let my bra straps show?

Yes, but only in certain situations, and you have to make it look purposeful. Bras with pretty, colorful straps can look like they were meant to peek out from under a tank top, while bras with worn-out, dirty straps do not. Don't ever let your straps show at work or school, but for shopping, dates, or a night out with friends, you have my endorsement to rock out with your straps out.

What about letting more of my bra show, like, through a sheer shirt? Is that cool? Or can I wear a bra as a shirt? Is that cool?

I hate imposing limits on the stylistic freedoms of my voluptuous sisters, but in general, smaller-chested ladies are able to show more skin without looking like harlots (but hey, if you're into the harlot look, then by all means). A black bra showing through a sheer shirt is a really cool look that a few lucky women are able to pull off with great success, but it's a tough style for the rest of us.

Less extreme versions of bra exhibitionism include letting a little lace peek out from under a simple tank top or showing pretty straps as described above. In general, wearing a bra as a shirt is not a good plan, as it can be quite chilly and is known to cause car accidents.

Cumulative Bra Knowledge Exam

Instructions—connect the type of bra in column A with the
article of clothing in column B it is best paired with:

Column A

1. Demi bra (a half-cup bra)

2. T-shirt bra (full-coverage
   bra in a soft fabric)

3. No bra

4. Strapless bra

5. Sports bra

6. Lacy bra

7. Nursing bra

Column B

A. Hippie halter top

B. Alma mater sweatshirt

C. Barf-stained "World's Best Mom"
   shirt

D. Low-cut tank top

E. T-shirt

F. Tube top

G. Pretty date dress

Answers: 1. D; 2. E; 3. A; 4. F; 5. B; 6. G; 7. C

Don't worry, if you didn't do so well on this test,
you'll have another chance in the underwear section. Your final
grade will be the average of your scores.

I am the proud owner of a serious rack. What kind of bra will keep me hoisted well above my belly button?

Oh, honey, do I feel ya. In general, if the bra meets two of the three following criteria, it will be able to handle your ample chest:

1. **Three or more hooks in the back**

2. **Wide, padded straps**

3. **Designed by NASA engineers**

My chest is, like, teeny tiny. Do I still have to wear a bra?

It depends on the sheerness of the shirt, the chill factor in the air, and your exhibitionist tendencies for the day. That being said, if I could go braless without risking great physical harm to myself and others, I would probably be like, "A bra? What's a bra?"

What about minimizers?

Here's the deal with minimizers: they're a good idea in theory. I mean, a magical bra that makes your breasts a full cup size smaller? Yes, please! But in practice, the things are usually bulky, uncomfortable, and bear a strong resemblance to nursing bras. Try them out and see what you think, but I'm going to stay maximized.

I haven't been feeling very good about myself lately. What should I do?

Buy a cute bra to make yourself feel better! What you wear under your clothes can have a huge effect on how you feel and the image and attitude you project to the world. Wear a sexy bra and panty set under your work clothes, school uniform, wet suit, whatever, and feel your mood change and your confidence soar.

FOR THE LOVE OF PANTIES

Interestingly enough, over the last fifty years or so, women's underwear options haven't changed all that drastically—the three mainstays are still basic briefs, kidney-crushing girdles, and shorts. Sure, thongs aren't just for strip clubs anymore, but I suppose we'll have to take that as proof of inevitable human progress.

What's great about underwear is that no matter your body's size or shape, you can find a style that's flattering on you and makes you feel good. I have friends who wear lacy thongs every day and friends who wear elastic-waist cotton briefs every day, and I can't detect a major difference in their levels of contentment. Wear whatever underwear feels right for you. My only stipulation: keep your panties in good working order. There's nothing worse for your self-image or love life than old, ratty underwear. Throw away your shabby pairs, and treat yourself to cute panties when you're feeling down. Trust me, it helps.

How Much to Spend

Don't spend too much on underwear. Unlike bras and construction cranes, a pair of underwear isn't hoisting anything up, so you can have more fun and focus less on quality. Love those $2 leopard print boyshorts on the clearance rack? Go for it. The $10 six-pack of cotton briefs sold at the big box store checkout? Totally fine.

To Match or Not to Match

Go to a lingerie boutique or open a bra catalog or watch a Halle Berry movie from the mid-'90s, and you're sure to be bombarded with sexy matching lingerie sets. These sets are often adorable and can cost more than a summer home in the Hamptons. So, should you spring for the matching bra and panties? Well, unless you are prepared to hire a private detective to track both parties' whereabouts, a matching lingerie set is just two pieces of clothing that will inevitably become separated. If you love each piece enough that you would have bought it on its own, then the set is worth it, but in my experience, that's not usually the case.

Sure, it's awesome when the stars align and both pieces of your matching lingerie set are clean and readily available to wear on the same day, but let's be honest—this will only happen a of couple times in your life, and matching sets can be spendy. Buy an assortment of black underwear instead—they're flattering, sexy, and will complement any bra you put on.

SHAPEWEAR

The word "shapewear" encompasses a world of undergarments, from slightly stretchy panties to spandex bodysuits tight enough to contain communism.

As someone who has always had an ample gut, I consider myself something of a shapewear connoisseur. I believe I have owned pretty much every undergarment ever claimed to slim and smooth a midsection. Sure, I could just tell you about my experiences and opinions, but that would be sort of boring for you and depressing for me, so read this thoroughly modernized fairy tale instead:

Goldilocks and the Three Tummy-Compressing Shapewear Options

Once upon a time, there was a gal named Goldilocks. Goldilocks was going to her friend's wedding. Goldilocks was a bridesmaid in said wedding and was being forced, completely against her will and good sense, to wear a revealing peachy pink slinky satin dress. If Goldilocks were to eat an egg sandwich and then put on this dress, passersby would be able to watch, in disturbing detail, as her breakfast traveled through the varying stages of digestion. Goldilocks sort of hated her friend at the moment, but that was OK, because she heard there were going to be some hot groomsmen and an open bar.

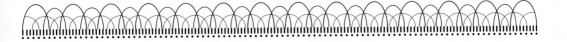

What Underwear to Wear, Where

All right, here's your chance to redeem a dreadful showing
on the bra quiz. Match the style of underwear
in the left column to its description on the right.

Column A

1. Briefs

2. Boyshorts

3. Thong

4. Supertight bodysuit

5. Girdle

Column B

A. No panty lines, constant wedgie

B. Everyday reliable

C. Flattering, sexy, adorable

D. Better left to our grandmothers

E. Confidence-boosting when
   you're wearing taffeta in front
   of four hundred people.

Answers: 1. B or C; 2. B or C; 3. A; 4. E; 5. D

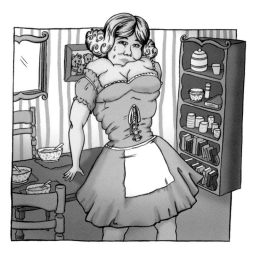

Walking down the street a few days before the wedding, Goldilocks passed a store that sold lingerie. She decided to go in, without bothering to check if it was owned by bears. Luckily it wasn't, and there, on the shelves, she found three styles of undergarments, all promising to shape and smooth her stomach.

Delighted, Goldilocks tried on the first option—a spandex bodysuit with a corseted waist and a built-in bra. "This is much too tight!" she gasped, "And it pushes all my stomach fat into my neck!" She wriggled out of it as quickly as possible. It took twenty minutes.

Goldilocks moved on to the second option—a nice pair of stretchy mid-rise panties. "These look comfortable," she said as she slipped them on. But they were much too loose! "You call these shapewear?" she asked mockingly, "I'm the same shape I was before!" She took them off.

Finally, she tried on the third option—a pair of panties with a lot of stretch, a thicker weave, and a high rise. "These go up past my belly button!" she giggled as she pulled them on, but she became silent when she looked in the mirror and saw her smooth, slim new tummy. "These are just right!" she declared, and decided to celebrate with an egg sandwich.

STYLE LESSON #14:

If you're in the market for shapewear, make like Goldilocks and find a style that's juuuuuust right: slimming undergarments should be tight enough to do the job, but not so tight that you can't bend at the waist.

How Much to Spend

Shapewear, since it serves an important purpose and is often infused with black magic and military-grade spandex, is more expensive than regular undergarments, but check out discount stores and sales for good deals. Here's a tongue twister for you: a slimming slip bought on sale slims just as well as a full-priced slimming slip. Say that three times fast, because it's true.

"I WEAR MY STAINED T-SHIRTS AT NIGHT," AND OTHER THINGS NOT TO DO

I believe that every woman should go to bed feeling beautiful. Yes, it sounds like an inspirational cliché, but I Googled it; it's not. This has been a personal creed of mine for some time for two reasons:

1. **If you go to bed dressed like a slobby sitcom husband,** it's that much harder to transform into a stylish, put-together woman in the morning.

2. **Pampering yourself before you go to bed** (especially if you're going to bed alone) is a reiteration that you're worth the effort, that looking and feeling good isn't a game you play for the world, it's for you.

So grab a pretty little nightgown in a soft fabric, or a cute tank top, or a matching flannel pajama set—just remember, whatever you wear to bed should make you feel like a million bucks. And that, my friends, is an inspirational cliché.

Nightwear and Relationships

Now, as wonderful as it is to feel beautiful at night purely for yourself, sometimes you want to feel beautiful for someone else, which brings us to the interesting realm of nightwear and relationships.

After doing extensive research, I have discovered that the inevitable relationship nightwear cycle is as follows:

THE BEGINNING: You excitedly frequent lingerie shops, picking out sexy unmentionables to debut under the covers.

THREE TO SIX MONTHS IN: You lose the sexy but uncomfortable unmentionables and switch to low-key but still flattering options, like a simple tank top and boyshorts.

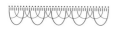

**FASHION RANT:
THE ROBE**

*I'm not a fan
of robes because I feel
they are the loungewear
equivalent of giving
up on life. Here's a challenge: put on a terrycloth
robe, and try to get
something accomplished.
I assure you that
you can't. No matter how
comfortable they may
be, traditional robes
are supremely unflatter-
ing and turn even the
most ambitious people
into particularly lazy
sloths. Harsh? Possibly,
but even though I've
only worn a robe a few
times in my life, I still
mourn the things
I didn't get done on
those days.*

THE END: You're stumbling into bed in questionable concert T-shirts, moaning, "Don't judge me!"

POST BREAKUP: You throw out the sexy unmentionables, chiding yourself for wasting your money on such foolish tokens of lust, but in the next relationship, the cycle begins anew, and you're back at the lingerie shop, asking about frequent shopper discounts.

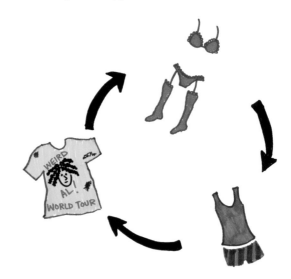

So, is there any respite from this madness? Yes, but in my experience, the only way to break the cycle is to bypass the beginning.

STYLE LESSON #15:

When it comes to dressing for bed while
in a relationship, start in the middle:
wear something flattering and sexy that's also
completely comfortable. If you avoid the
lace teddies, hopefully you will not be tempted
into the sad nightwear graveyard of
Weird Al World Tour T-shirts.

Ribbed tank tops and boyshorts are always cute, or you could try pretty briefs and a fitted T-shirt, or maybe a short nightgown in a practical fabric, like cotton. Make an effort, but not so much of an effort that you can't maintain the standard. And whether you go to bed alone or with a suitor, always wear something you love.

TIGHTS ARE TIGHT!
("TIGHT," HERE, MEANING COOL)

Socks, tights, nylons, and eight-tracks: two of these items have been almost completely phased out of modern day life. Can you guess which ones?

That's right. Nylons and eight-tracks. These prehistoric relics might be good for some reminiscing and a laugh, but for the most part, it comes down to this: if you want to listen to music in today's world, you use an MP3 player, and if you want to cover your legs, you wear tights. Get a pair of control top tights in a color you love, and you'll reap all the benefits of nylons without the dramatic aging effect.

Speaking of Tights . . .

I adore black tights. They're flattering and versatile and kind of keep you warm (well, that's what I always told my dad when he demanded to know why I was wearing a miniskirt and tights in December instead of his highly recommended flannel-lined L.L.Bean jeans). Everything, including flannel-lined L.L.Bean jeans, looks better with a pair of black tights.

While black tights have the power to add a dose of chic to any outfit, brightly colored tights are another favorite of mine for their ability to add a dose of funky. If a nun added bright pink tights to her habit, she would look so funky and cool that everyone would start asking her where she got her outfit; and she would say "God," and then things would get sort of uncomfortable.

If you've never played with colored tights, entering this new realm of accessories can be a bit daunting. See "Handy Guide to Hosiery Pairings" on the next page if you'd like some extra help.

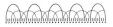

NOTABLE EXEMPTIONS TO MY NO-ROBE RULE:

1.
You have the flu.

2.
You are at the hospital.

3.
It is Christmas morning.

4.
Your robe is short and made of pretty silk.

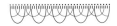

HANDY GUIDE TO HOSIERY PAIRINGS

COLOR	DESCRIPTION	SUGGESTED PAIRINGS
Red tights	Bold, intense, full-bodied	Denim skirt, black blazer
White tights	Crisp, dry, self-esteem draining	Zero body fat
Black tights	Slightly oaky, flattering, versatile, chic	EVERYTHING
Navy blue tights	Rich, smooth, conservative, stylish	Brown shoes. No, white shoes. Wait, no. Help!
Printed tights	Spicy, daring, fashion forward, hip	Simple, monochromatic outfits
Neon tights (variety of colors)	Intense bouquet, funky	Dresses and boots; '80s parties
Fishnet tights	Complex, sexy, infuriating to put on	Layered over colored tights
Green tights	Earth-scented, tricky	Praying mantis costume

Shopping for tights, like shopping for sunglasses (see Chapter 8), divides people into Disposers and Investors. The difference is that while it's possible for a pair of sunglasses to last five years or more (I said possible, not probable), a pair of tights just won't.

I've always thought that paying more for designer tights is like paying more for designer paint colors. I have yet to hear of someone walking into a friend's kitchen and exclaiming, "Oh! What a lovely shade of white! Is that Ralph Lauren?" Similarly, I've never seen a pair of generic black tights and thought, "Calvin Klein has done it again!"

STYLE LESSON #16:

Spend enough on tights so that they'll last for more than one wearing, but not so much that you'll feel like a fool when they die (because they will die, probably soon).

Yes, I'm something of a hosiery nihilist, but I'm a perky nihilist with helpful tips! Behold:

➤ **TO EXTEND THE LIVES OF YOUR TIGHTS,** go for the thickest pairs possible, the ones that could aaaalllmooossst double as pants.

➤ **TREAT YOUR TIGHTS LIKE A BABY:** hand wash them in lukewarm sink baths and sing them lullabies at night.

➤ **WHEN YOU PUT YOUR TIGHTS ON,** do so slowly and with care so as not to scratch them.

I've heard legends from faraway lands of tights lasting as long as five years, but I believe my personal record is two years.

Ways to Wear Tights

While socks with sandals is, of course, a big no-no (I think that's in the Bible), I love the look of bright tights with open-toed shoes in the winter. You have to wear it like you really mean it, but if you do, it's a great way to get more mileage out of your warm weather footwear.

Footless tights are a fun addition to any hosiery wardrobe. Try them in an unexpected color, and wear them with at least a bit of a heel, as their cropped nature can make legs look stumpy. They're especially great tucked into boots.

If you love the look of kneesocks but don't enjoy looking like a schoolgirl, not to worry—with numerous nonschoolgirl precautions, it's possible to pull this style off. Go for options with grown-up details or designs, like lace insets or dark colors, and let your socks peek out of winter boots or wedge heels. Avoid pairing with little oxford shoes and plaid miniskirts at all costs.

IT'S WHAT'S UNDER
YOUR CLOTHES THAT COUNTS

It's easy to assume that until scientists perfect X-ray vision, what you wear under your clothes is inconsequential, but this just isn't true. Not only do undergarments affect how your clothing fits, they can affect (and reflect) your mood, confidence level, and even the state of your relationship. Everyone knows you should dress for the job you want; a lesser known truth is that you should wear undergarments for the life you want.

So put some thought into which bra and underwear you put on today. Try a daring new style of hosiery. Throw away the unflattering XL T-shirt you always end up wearing to bed. Seriously, make some minor changes to your undergarment routine and see what a difference it makes. In the meantime, repeat after me: "A good foundation is essential. A good foundation is essential. A good foundation is essential. . . . "

FIVE

From Ankle Straps to Zippers:

AN A–Z GUIDE TO ALL THINGS SHOE

SHOES ARE OBVIOUSLY ONE OF THE GREATEST INNOVATIONS in human history; after all, high heels are what separate us from the apes. I love shoes because they're a fun, stylish way to express yourself and, as an added benefit, they protect your feet from hot concrete and infectious hypodermic needles.

Like many of you out there, I've been a fan of interesting, eye-catching shoes for as long as I can remember. One day in the fourth grade, I even wore one purple Keds sneaker and one pink Keds sneaker to match my purple and pink plaid dress; my teacher swiftly and without explanation placed me in a special needs class. This creative-footwear persecution did nothing to stifle my passion, and today I'm the proud owner of many pairs of beautiful shoes in all colors of the rainbow (although I do usually try to match them up).

The world of footwear is so wide-ranging and exciting that I thought it best to present this chapter in a rigid A–Z format for ease of reference. Here you'll find every fact and figure I've discovered—every tip, anecdote, and observation I've ever had—about those glorious things called shoes.

A IS FOR ANKLE STRAP

Shoes with straps across the ankles are perhaps the most maligned footwear of the twenty-first century, with the possible exception of plastic clogs. Ask anyone, from a powerful fashion editor to a line cook at IHOP, and you'll hear the same sentiments: ankle straps are evil! Ankle straps make your legs look fat! Ankle straps were the second shooter on the grassy knoll!

As with most matters of style, however, I take a less extreme viewpoint. I believe the ankle strap is sort of like the really tall, thin, pretty girl in your high school class—sure, she's intimidating, and standing next to her makes you look short and frumpy, but if you get to know her, she's not that bad.

Here's the thing: if you find shoes you absolutely love, and they happen to have ankle straps, I don't think that fact should warrant an automatic reshelve. Try them on. Do they make your legs look like sausages stuffed into too-small casings? If so, you should probably put the shoes back; but if not, here are a couple tips to help you conquer an acute fear of ankle straps:

➤ **TRY TIGHTS.** Opaque tights, especially black ones, make legs look so long and lean that unflattering shoes hardly matter. Tights the same color as your shoes = legs for miles, ankle straps or not.

➤ **IF YOU LOVE THE SHOES** except for the ankle straps, wear them with slim pants that show everything but the offending straps.

➤ **THE HIGHER AND THE THICKER THE HEELS,** the longer and slimmer your legs look. This rule applies to all shoes, but it's especially applicable when considering ankle straps. There's a much greater chance that four-inch platforms with ankle straps will look fabulous on you than flat shoes with ankle straps.

➤ **SPEAKING OF FLAT SHOES WITH ANKLE STRAPS**—the likelihood of these looking amazing hovers at about 2 percent. Seriously, you didn't hear it from me, but I heard flat shoes with ankle straps actually killed Elvis. Proceed with caution.

B IS FOR BOOTS

In all my years of doling out fashion advice, by far the most frequently asked questions have been about boots. Here are some of the most frequent frequently asked questions:

I love the look of jeans tucked into boots, but I'm not sure how to pull it off. Any advice?

I love this look too, and pulling it off is actually less about the boots and more about the jeans. Few things look worse than baggy, bunched-up jeans haphazardly shoved into a nice pair of boots. If you're a fan of the jeans-tucked-into-boots look, it's worth purchasing some super skinny, tapered jeans that may be completely unflattering sans boots but look fabulous and polished when tucked in. Dark, slim-fitting jeans are great with most boot options. Try tucking jeans into basic riding boots for a preppy, equestrian-inspired look, or opt for motorcycle boots to up your badass quotient.

My calves are HUGE—like, next to me, a rhino's legs look dainty—can I ever enjoy boots like a normal person?

Of course you can! The search may be a bit harder (and by "a bit harder," I mean you may want to rip the too-tight boots off and hurl them at the salespeople, screaming, "WHO could actually wear these?"), but with some shopping endurance and creativity, I assure you that everyone can find boots that work for them. First, try a store that focuses on plus size clothing. Even if the rest of you isn't plus sized, those stores may carry accessories (read: boots!) in adjusted sizing that will work for you. Next, broaden your search to online retailers. Specialty shoe Web sites often include whole categories dedicated to wide calf boots. Order a few pairs online and send back the ones that don't work. And finally, if you find the perfect pair but they're a little snug, have a cobbler stretch them for you. Like Jesus turned water into wine, cobblers can turn too-tight boots into your new favorite footwear.

And the opposite problem:

My feet and calves are so tiny that boots don't fit me right. What do I do?

Definitely look online, because those specialty shoe Web sites have narrow calf categories too. Also, try the kids' section. Seriously. Have you seen how stylish preteen girls are these days? If you're especially petite, check out the kids' section at a high-end department store for shoes and boots that are stylish, cheaper than their "adult" counterparts, and actually fit you correctly. I won't tell.

Is it possible to wear ankle boots without looking like a stump?

Yes. Even though they can be shockingly unflattering, ankle boots are so undeniably cool that they're worth giving a try. The tips I mentioned for ankle straps also apply to ankle boots: the higher the heel, the better, and try pairing them with dark, opaque tights or slim pants.

My big, fuzzy sheepskin boots are soooo comfy! Are they really a fashion no-no?

Listen, the fashion bullies have obviously never tried on big, fuzzy sheepskin boots. Maybe don't wear them to work or to defend your thesis, but for cozy weekends—absolutely. Try them with tucked-in jeans or with thick tights and skirts.

The only reason I have a job is so I can wear cute boots to work in the fall and winter. Is that weird?

Not at all.

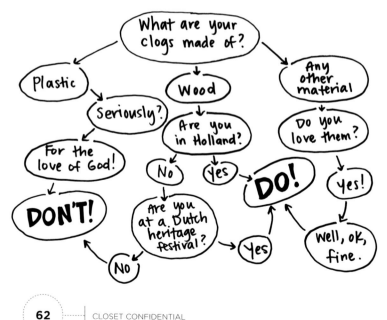

C IS FOR CLOGS

Wondering if that pair of clogs is a "Do" or a "Don't"? Consult this handy flowchart to find out!

D IS FOR DON'T GET PRESSURED INTO BUYING $1,000 SHOES

Go to a top-of-the-line department store or a luxury Web site, or open a fashion magazine, and you will find designer shoes that cost $1,000, sometimes more. At the risk of agreeing with my father, I think this is insane. Everyone loves to splurge every once in a while, but if I have the choice between a pair of cute heels and a round-trip ticket to Europe, I'll get on the plane to Italy barefoot. As much as I love shoes, I believe there are more important things in life, and I also believe you can procure really good shoes for around $100 (and top designer shoes on sale for around $300).

The problem is, if you follow fashion at all, you're going to encounter tremendous pressure to spend four-digit sums of money on designer shoes. Fashion magazines, Web sites, TV shows, and maybe even your friends will try to convince you that those lime green Givenchy platforms are totally worth it, and it can be hard to say no.

When I was in the sixth grade, my school had a program called "Just Say No" that placed portly, retired police officers in the classroom to teach us how to resist when big-city drug dealers invaded the playground and offered us narcotics. One of the techniques our portly cop employed was role-playing, during which one student would play a drug dealer and the other would awkwardly practice saying no to scripted offers of methamphetamines and crack cocaine. I would inevitably be paired up with the dreamiest boy in class and have to say things like, "No thanks, dude! Why would I need drugs to have fun when I could play my Super Nintendo instead?"

Although I read later that the "Just Say No" program did nothing but create more effective drug dealers (I guess the kids playing the bad guys took their roles pretty seriously), I think we can apply this technique to the peer pressure surrounding expensive designer shoes.

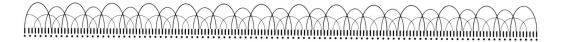

Just Say No to $1,000 Shoes!

Role-play the following situations with a friend to learn to resist the pressure.

SCENARIO #1:

Big-City Designer Shoe Dealer: Hey, you should buy this pair of Christian Louboutin peep-toe pumps! They're $900, but they'll make you forget all your problems and feel high as a kite!

You: No thank you, dude. (Firmly) I do not need shoes to make me feel good about life! Well, sometimes I do, but I will get my kicks on sale. Thank you.

SCENARIO #2:

Big-City Designer Shoe Dealer: Hey, even though these five-inch platform heels are $850, it's totally worth it because they're soooooo comfortable!

You: Ha, nice try (laugh nonchalantly), but you can't fool me. Five-inch heels, whether they are $30 or $3,000, are about as comfortable as a gynecological exam.

SCENARIO #3:

Big-City Designer Shoe Dealer: Hey, I know you're hesitant about spending so much on shoes, but look, I've created this little chart that shows you exactly why designer shoes cost so much, and it makes perfect sense! Ostrich skin doesn't come cheap, you know!

You: Hmm . . . (stroke chin as if in thought) Tempting . . . but even if you can justify it, that doesn't make it right!

Now, if these exercises are as effective as my school's "Just Say No" program, within the next five years you should be working as a successful drug dealer.

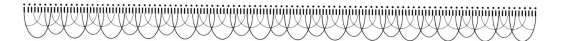

E IS FOR EVERY WOMAN SHOULD HAVE THE FOLLOWING SHOES IN HER CLOSET

ABSOLUTE MUST-HAVES:

➤ **A comfortable pair of black mid-height heels** (for work and dates/weekend)

➤ **Cute flats** (for anytime)

➤ **Quality boots** that get better with age (for work/weekend/play)

➤ **A pair of pretty sandals** for summer (flip-flops only count if you're a professional surfer)

➤ **Dressy shoes** (for formal occasions—can be cheap and uncomfortable if you're low on funds, but a nice, comfortable pair is always good to own)

➤ **Sneakers** (for the gym)

USEFUL ADD-ONS:

➤ **Two to twenty more pairs** of any of the shoes listed above (a girl's gotta have some variety in her life)

➤ **Wedge heels** (for work and play)

➤ **Platform heels** (for glamour)

➤ **Cute, non-gym sneakers** (for weekends or trips with lots of walking)

➤ **Another pair of boots** (for work/weekend/play)

➤ **Flip-flops** (for weekends and the beach)

FUN ADD-ONS:

➤ **Giant, cozy snow boots** (for casual winter days)

➤ **Crazy, expensive, eye-catching high heels** that elicit stares and strong opinions (for making an entrance)

➤ **Moccasins** (for running errands and trips to Alaska)

F IS FOR FLATS

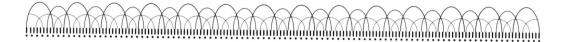

Why I Love Flats: A Short, Passionate Essay

Flat shoes are my favorite thing in the world. I love them more than pandas and milkshakes combined. If I die prematurely, it will probably be from being crushed under my massive pile of ballet flats. Flats are comfortable and chic, and they come in many styles that are just as exciting and eye catching as heels (my current favorite pair are bright orange satin with a fist-sized fabric flower affixed to the toe of each). Plus, Jackie O. and Audrey Hepburn favored them. Do you want to argue with Jackie O. and Audrey Hepburn? No? Good.

G IS FOR GO TO THE STORE
AND BUY SOME BALLET FLATS

Yeah, I'm pretty serious about this.

H IS FOR HEELS

While I've made no secret of my preference for flats, that doesn't mean I don't love good heels. Heels are capable of wonderful feats, like making you three inches taller and slimming your legs and allowing too-long pants to fit perfectly. Here's a more specific breakdown of different types of heels and their pros and cons:

Kitten Heel

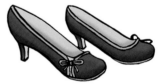

Pros: Cute and dainty

Cons: Can make legs look distinctly un-dainty by comparison

Wedge Heel

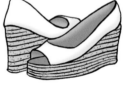

Pros: Funky, fashionable, and usually more comfortable than regular heels

Cons: Can be weighty and cumbersome

Low Heel (1 inch or lower)

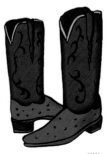

Pros: Comfortable and reasonable

Cons: Can look, hmm—how do I put this?—comfortable and reasonable

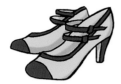

Mid-Height Heel (1½–2½ inches)

Pros: Comfortable and flattering

Cons: Many mid-height shoe styles are sort of boring

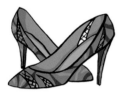

High Heel
(3 inches or higher)

Pros: Glamorous and fashion forward

Cons: Can be painful

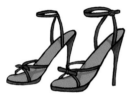

Stiletto Heel

Pros: Sexy, can be used as a weapon if necessary

Cons: A pencil-width heel supporting your entire body mass is not going to be especially comfortable

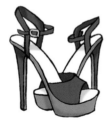

Super-High Heel
(5 inches or higher)

Pros: Umm . . . they make you five inches taller?

Cons: Chances of tripping and breaking your ankle: 95 percent

I IS FOR IF YOU'RE WEARING COLORFUL RAIN BOOTS, A MONSOON IS NOTHING BUT AN EXCUSE TO SPLASH THROUGH PUDDLES

Rain boots have recently come back into style, and I couldn't be happier. These waterproof miracles blend fashion and function so as to make it possible for grown women to jump in mud puddles.

The key to wearing rain boots is to accept and embrace the fact that you're going to look like a six-year-old from the knee down and to compensate from the knee up. For example, the day you wear your bright pink rain boots may not be the best day to wear your yellow coat with fuzzy ears attached to the hood, or your rainbow candy necklace. Try colorful rain boots with black slacks and a classic trench coat instead, or with black tights and a dress. Stow respectable work shoes in your tote bag so you can still sport those yellow polka dot boots on your way to the office, and soon you'll be saying, "Daily grind? What daily grind? I got to splash around in puddles this morning!"

J IS FOR JUMP AROUND IN YOUR SHOES BEFORE YOU BUY THEM

You never know when the need to frolic will arise, so it's imperative that you be prepared. This is more useful (and fun) than walking sedately around the shoe store. You probably did this when you were a kid; why did you stop?

K IS FOR KNOW YOUR FRIENDS' SHOE SIZES

So, say you're at a vintage store and come across the most amazing, gorgeous, pristine gold Gucci heels from the '70s for $20, but there's a problem: The shoes are a size 10. You're a size 7. It doesn't matter. Whatever. You try them on, walk around in them, and of course they slip off and look generally bad. Other shoppers notice how amazing they are and start to hover like hungry vintage vultures. You're sweating now, racking your brain, thinking, "Is there a procedure that's, like, the opposite of foot binding, that makes your feet bigger?" You realize your thoughts make you sound like an idiot, and of course there's no such procedure, and even if there was you would never be that shallow, except you totally would be because these shoes are AMAZING. The vintage vultures are closing in. Oh my God, what are you going to do?!

Here's what you do: You remember that your friend Katelyn wears a size 10. You buy the shoes for her. You earn good shoe karma and peace of mind knowing that the shoes will have a warm, loving home. Bonus: Next time your friend Katelyn tries and fails to squeeze into a size 7 pair of vintage riding boots, she'll think of you.

L IS FOR LIMPING

On any city sidewalk, at any given moment, there is a woman limping along, grimacing, and trying to maintain an air of sexy nonchalance. There's a good chance that this woman is me. For as much as I know about shoes, and how many shoes I've worn, and how much shoe advice I've dispensed, I still fall into the uncomfortable shoe trap on a fairly regular basis.

STYLE LESSON #17:

For many women, limping around in uncomfortable shoes is akin to childbirth: in the midst of it, you're in extraordinary pain, cursing under your breath and vowing that you will never go through this again. But as soon as you get home, you forget about all the agony and the blood; you see those cute little shoes sitting there looking so harmless and helpless and suddenly you're putting them on and going through the same thing all over again.

We must try to overcome this vicious cycle for the sake of our poor feet and sanities. I've found that going shopping with a brother, father, boyfriend, husband, or male therapist is a good deterrent, because they will inevitably say, as you slip on those studded stilettos, "Those CAN'T be comfortable!" Unfortunately, I tend to choose the shoes over the man mocking the shoes, but it's a good plan in theory.

M IS FOR MULE

The word "mule" can be used to describe an open-backed shoe or a South American pack animal; confusing the two could prove disastrous. Check out this chart for easy identification.

CHARACTERISTIC	TRANSPORTS WATER THROUGH ANDES MOUNTAINS	LOOKS AWKWARD WITH HOSIERY	EXCELLENT TRACTION ON CLAY SOILS	RESISTANT TO SUN AND MOISTURE	MAKES A CLOMPING SOUND WHEN WALKING	INTOLERANT OF DOGS
Mule (shoe)		X			X	X
Mule (pack animal)	X	X	X	X	X	X

N IS FOR NEVER VISIT A FOREIGN COUNTRY WITHOUT KNOWING HOW TO SAY "SHOE"

Any number of circumstances could precipitate the need to buy shoes in a strange land, from having your sandal devoured by piranhas in Brazil to spotting an amazing pair of stilettos in the window of an Italian boutique. Being prepared for such situations just makes sense. Here is a handy guide to useful translations of the word "shoe":

Spanish: *zapato*

French: *chaussure*

German: *schuh*

Swedish: *sko*

Italian: *scarpa*

Portuguese: *sapato*

Japanese: *hannaga*

Farsi: *kafsh*

Swahili: *kiatu*

Women buy and wear hot shoes for other women. We should all just accept this, and embrace this, and be happy.

O IS FOR "OH MY GOD! I LOVE YOUR SHOES!" AND OTHER THINGS A MAN WILL NEVER SAY TO YOU

If you still saunter through the shoe section looking for the perfect high heels to impress your man, or the ultimate strappy sandals to score you a hottie at the club, trust me, some day you'll see the light. You'll be sitting in the coffee shop wearing some impossibly expensive high heels, and the 4,000th woman in a row will tap you on the shoulder and say, "Oh my God! I love your shoes!" and you'll sigh and give her a half-assed "Thanks," while staring longingly at the hot guy a few tables over for whom the expensive high heels were intended and who is not complimenting your shoes (and will never compliment your shoes). Then it hits you: here you are, waiting and yearning for the male attention you dreamed your footwear would bring, brushing off all these perfectly lovely female compliments. But what if those female compliments are good enough? What if they're better than good? Why are 4,000 women's compliments not as good as one man's?

Let me tell you, they're much better. Getting a shoe compliment from a woman is like having Ina Garten come up to you at a party and tell you your seven-layer dip is incredible; like having Whitney Houston tap on your car window at a stoplight and tell you that she overheard your rendition of "I Will Always Love You" and that you've really got something there; like having Mario Testino tap you on the shoulder when you're taking MySpace pictures in front of your bathroom mirror and saying, "You've got a good eye, kid." We women know our shoes, and our compliments should be appreciated and savored accordingly.

This is not to discount male shoe appreciation entirely. Some men are very knowledgeable about shoes, and even those who aren't sometimes make an effort: my boyfriend will throw me a "nice shoes" bone every once in a while. But the truth is, if I put him in front of a shoe lineup that included a pair of ballet flats, some high heels, some nice boots, a pair of sandals, and those giant, clunky, thigh-high leg braces that Forrest Gump had to wear as a child, and I asked, "Which footwear seen here do I NOT wear regularly?" he'd sweat and crack his knuckles and squint and finally break down and scream, "Good God! Lay off! I have no idea!"

Think about it: How many times in your life has a man complimented you on your shoes? A few? Four, five, ten if you're lucky? Now, how many times in your life has a man asked you, "Why the heck do you need so many shoes?" Yeah, that's what I thought.

P IS FOR PRACTICE WALKING IN HEELS

I know you've heard this about a billion times, but that's because it's really good advice. One of the many things that can kill a fabulous outfit is teetering around awkwardly on heels you're not sure how to walk in. Looking natural and graceful in heels is an acquired art: you have to work at it.

I have a friend who wears heels everyday and walks around as if she is floating on air. I asked her for her secret, expecting a cute story about walking around in her mother's heels when she was a kid, or a lie about how it's always come naturally for her. Instead, she told me that when she was fourteen, she worked in a boutique that was frequented by a group of drag queens. These fairy godfathers took her under their sequined wings and taught her a number of priceless lessons, like how to apply false eyelashes and how to walk in heels. "You are the luckiest girl in the world," I told her, and I meant it.

STYLE LESSON #19:

If you can find a band of kindly drag queens
to teach you how to walk in heels,
then good for you, but if you're not that lucky,
practice on your own.

High Heels How-To for Those of Us without Drag Queen Tutors

➤ **STAND UP STRAIGHT** (balance is key) and take smaller steps than usual. If you're going to wear high heels, you must accept that your pace will be slowed considerably, which is fine—you'll always be *fashionably* late.

➤ **PUT YOUR HEEL DOWN FIRST** with each step, then your toe. Continue this pattern. Don't clomp around like a horse.

➤ **IF YOU'RE STILL TEETERING,** try placing each foot directly ahead of the other, as if you were walking on a balance beam.

➤ **WALK FORCEFULLY AND CONFIDENTLY;** don't fight the exaggerated swing of your hips, which is part of the appeal of high heels.

➤ **PRACTICE, PRACTICE, PRACTICE.** Wear your heels around the house, to the store, to play basketball, and in no time your high-heeled walk will look less accident-waiting-to-happen and more chic and natural.

Q IS FOR QUALITY

When it comes to shoes, quality counts. It's cliché and boring, and it sucks because those pink pleather pumps are soooooo cute, but it's true: cheap, poorly made shoes are the devil's work (little-known fact: the devil deals mostly in blisters and foot and back pain. Also see "L Is for Limping"). Quality shoes don't have to be extremely expensive or designer. Look for the following features to help spot superior shoes:

➤ **Genuine leather or other fabrics with some give and flexibility**

➤ **Padded insoles**

➤ **Fully lined insides**

➤ **Sturdy heels**

➤ **Firmly attached details (such as buckles)**

R IS FOR THE REASON WE LOVE SHOES

I've scoured seven continents, consulted with the world's top psychologists, physicists, and astrologists, read every holy book, and graduated from Harvard Law with a PhD in shoe-ology, all to figure out why women love shoes so much, and now, for the first time, I'm going to share my findings with the world:

Shoes Fit, Even On Fat Days

So, there you go.

S IS FOR SNEAKER

Remember how, under "A," I proved my shoe tolerance by defending ankle straps? Then, under "B," I even approved big, fuzzy sheepskin boots? Well, one footwear scenario for which I have significantly less patience is when athletic shoes are worn outside of an exercise situation. Perhaps I'm jaded after growing up fifteen miles from Nike's headquarters, in the casual Northwest, where grungy sneakers are more common than high heels, but I mourn the adorable outfits that have been marred by out-of-context sneakers. It's very difficult to make running shoes fashionable, especially if they're used regularly for running, which guarantees they're dirty and noticeably worn.

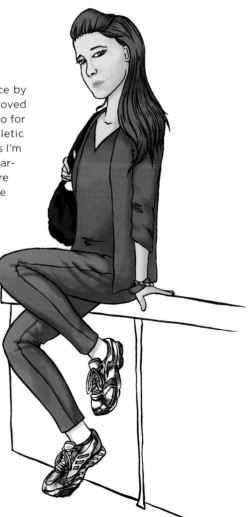

ALTERNATIVES TO PETROLEUM	ALTERNATIVES TO GRUNGY SNEAKERS
Biodiesel	Ballet flats (see "F")
Ethanol	Moccasins
Nuclear power	Flat sandals
Wind power	Low-heeled boots
Solar/wave power	Cute, clean, not-for-the-gym sneakers

T IS FOR TOE

Round toes, pointy toes, peep-toes, square toes—it can be hard to keep these different shoe styles straight! Here's a nursery rhyme that might help:

Those round-toe pumps are retro cool
and look good on all the ladies,

While square toes—
sorry, I'm being honest—
should have been left in the '80s.

Want longer legs?
Try a pointy toe;
it'll lengthen your gams by a mile,

But don't go too pointy,
or you'll look like a witch,
and witches are rarely in style.

Peep-toes are great for summer,
but in winter watch out for frostbite,

Better yet, to stay stylish and warm,
pair your open-toed shoes with bright tights.

U IS FOR UNIQUE

Shoes are a fun and easy way to show off your unique style without risking your job or reputation. So be bold! Be daring! Wear colors on your feet that you would never wear on your chest. Pair leopard print stilettos with basic black office wear. Get a pair of clunky, scuffed-up boots and wear them with a flouncy sundress. Use your shoes to express yourself, because life is too short for boring footwear.

V IS FOR VINTAGE

I consider vintage shopping to be one of the greatest joys of the mortal world, and a huge part of the appeal is searching for old, awesome shoes. I scour thrift stores, estate sales, vintage boutiques, and auction Web sites looking for great deals on glamorous shoes that have been around longer than me, and I've been rewarded with a number of brag-worthy finds. Still, I completely understand many people's hesitation—after all, "vintage shoes" is a nice way of saying "old, previously worn shoes," which is sort of unappealing. Here are a few tips that help make the experience more pleasant, because I swear, it's worth it:

➤ **WEAR HOSIERY.** Stepping barefoot into a twenty-year-old boot can be frightening. A layer of nylon helps.

➤ **LOOK FOR VINTAGE SHOES** in fair condition for $20 or less, but think about spending more for vintage shoes that still look new: if they've lasted this long, they'll probably outlast the human race.

➤ **REMEMBER, YOU CAN ALWAYS TAKE VINTAGE SHOES** to a cobbler to have nasty soles replaced and heels reinforced. You can also spray the heck out of your new treasures with disinfectant for a nicer smell and peace of mind.

➤ **HAVE YOUR DREAM VINTAGE SHOES IN MIND** when shopping, but be open to other possibilities. I've been looking for some perfectly worn-in '70s riding boots for about half my life, but in the meantime I've found '80s platforms, '60s sandals, and '50s peep-toe pumps.

➤ **IF THE THRILL OF THE HUNT** (and the trying on of old shoes) isn't your thing, just shop vintage and auction Web sites instead. Usually you'll pay more, but you get to sort through better-quality merchandise.

W IS FOR WHAT SHOES DO I WEAR WITH . . .

JEANS?

Flats, heels, wedges, boots, or sandals. (For more information, see the "Denim Field Guide" in Chapter 1.)

WORK PANTS?

Mid-height pumps, dressy flats, short wedges, ankle boots, or high heels if you don't have to walk too much.

A DRESS?

Any height heels, flats, wedges, sandals, or boots. (Tough, worn-in boots with a feminine dress are always a stylish choice.)

CROPPED PANTS?

Ballet flats for a cute, retro look; sandals; or mid-height heels. Definitely not ankle boots, unless you're trying to make your legs look about a foot shorter.

A MINISKIRT?

Flats, low wedges, low- or mid-height heels, kitten heels, sandals, or boots. Always remember this simple equation: high heels + short skirt = up to no good.

CUTOFFS?

Cute sneakers (see "S Is for Sneaker" for guidelines), sandals, wedges, or flats.

X IS FOR X-RAY

Have you ever seen an A–Z list that didn't have "X-ray" for X? Yeah, me neither.

Y IS FOR YEARNING

If you really, really love a pair of shoes, and they don't cost $1,000, you should get them. So what if your friends wouldn't be caught dead in puffy pink snow boots, or every fashion magazine tells you that ankle boots will make you look slightly squatter than an Oompa Loompa? If a pair of shoes takes your breath away, and you can't get them out of your head, and especially if they go on sale, you should get them.

STYLE LESSON #20:

You can work pretty much any shoes into your style and wardrobe with a little creativity, and if all else fails, just put them on a shelf above your bed and enjoy sweet shoe dreams for life.

Z IS FOR ZIPPERS

Look for details like studs, zippers, unique textures, grommets, laces, bows, and straps to set your shoes apart or, to really make an entrance, find shoes that incorporate all of these elements. I once saw a woman walking down the street wearing platform sandals that seemed to be constructed entirely of metal studs and zippers. I'm not really sure how they stayed on her feet, or how she kept from wincing in pain, but I will never forget those shoes.

Well, there you have it. A comprehensive guide to ~~all~~ most things shoe. If you take anything away from this chapter, let it not be a newfound knowledge of pack mules, but an excitement and fearlessness about footwear. Shoes are such a great excuse to make bold style choices, so try something new. Excluding severe bunions, there's really no reason not to strut your stuff in some sexy high heels, or splash around in floral-patterned rain boots. Wear your personality on your feet, and you'll walk with your head held high.

SIX

The Bags We Carried:

THE PRACTICAL, PHILOSOPHICAL, AND FASHIONABLE IMPLICATIONS OF A WOMAN'S PURSE

CALL ME MELODRAMATIC (you wouldn't be the first today), but I think a purse is so much more than a black hole in which to lose your keys. A purse, more than any other accessory or item of clothing, is laden with deep emotional and personal implications. Our handbags are microcosms of our lives—to take a peek inside a woman's purse is to see an intimate snapshot of her world. In my first creative writing class my freshman year of college, my teacher, a pretentious, ponytailed male grad student, told us to empty our pockets or purses and write about the contents. When I dumped my purse out onto the desk—actually, it took two desks to hold the aggregate mass—my classmates found out that I carry one dirty sock (That's right. Not two. One.) and enough tampons to last me until menopause. To spite my teacher for putting me through such a traumatic exposé, I penned a free verse poem about the dirty sock instead of writing the normal expository paragraph about the contents of my purse. He gave me a D.

These days, I'm older and wiser, so no more dirty socks in the purse for me! Aside from my wallet, here's a list of the necessities in my purse right now:

➤ **A stick of Japanese gum my brother bought online**

➤ **One puka seashell**

➤ **Enough energy bars to feed a small village** (all with one bite out of them—I always forget that they're gross)

➤ **Approximately seven hundred bobby pins**

➤ **A map of the Pacific Islands**

➤ **String cheese. Old string cheese. Oh my God.**

➤ **A notebook**

➤ **Pens**

➤ **Old lip balm with sand in it**

➤ **A Catholic prayer card** (I'm not Catholic)

➤ **Every receipt I've amassed since 2003**

➤ **One of those miniature pencils from a bowling alley**

➤ **A lollipop**

What's that you say? None of these items are necessary at all? Well, what if I'm walking down the street and run into an extremely attractive singer-songwriter who's freaking out because he has a great idea for a hit song but doesn't have a writing utensil handy? I simply reach into my purse and give him a pen and notebook, which he uses to scribe his hit tune. He's so grateful that he wants to serenade me, but as he opens his mouth, his dry lips crack! "Lip balm with sand in it?" I ask, handing it over to him. After using it, he smacks his lips, marveling aloud at the combination of moisture and exfoliation. "Moisture *and* exfoliation?" a passing entrepreneur exclaims, "I think you're onto something there! Would you like my help marketing sandy lip balm as the next must-have cosmetic?" I say, "Of course!" to which the entrepreneur replies, "We must go to the Pacific Islands immediately to harvest the finest sand! If only we had a map . . . " "Don't worry about that," I say, and bidding adieu to the attractive singer-songwriter (leaving him with a lollipop to remember me by), I head to the airport with the entrepreneur.

Soon after our plane takes off, we run into trouble—one of the wings is falling off! The pilot screams over the intercom, "Does anyone have a powerful adhesive? American gum would be too weak, but perhaps Japanese gum would work! Does anyone have any Japanese gum?" I seize the gum from my purse and slide it up the aisle to the pilot, who begins to repair the wing. "Please pray for us!" the flight attendant begs the priest sitting next to me, but he's too frozen with fear to act! Luckily, I have my prayer card in my purse and lead everyone in an impromptu Catholic mass. The pilot then comes into the cabin, looking grim. "The wing is repaired, but I forgot to put cheese on my salami sandwich." With a wink and a smile, I toss him my moldy string cheese, which he declares perfectly aged and a delicious contrast with the salty cured meat. Crisis averted!

Finally, we arrive at our destination—a remote island in the Pacific. As the entrepreneur and I begin gathering sand, we find ourselves face-to-face with an angry tribe of indigenous pygmies. Through a series of hand signals, the chief tells us that we may take sand, but we must offer something in return. "How about energy bars?" I suggest. "I have enough for the whole village!" The tribe rejoices and as they eat, the entrepreneur hands them a contract. By signing it, they receive 20 percent of the profits from our sandy lip balm. They love this idea, but the entrepreneur's pens are too big for their tiny hands! I dig through my purse and find the miniature pencil—perfect. We're ready to leave now, but I want to buy a souvenir to remember my time on the island. Unfortunately, the tribal store doesn't take Visa. "How much for the shrunken head?" I ask. The tribal store clerk tells me it costs one puka seashell. "No problem," I say, giving him the one I've been carrying in my handbag for three years. We say good-bye to our new friends and get on a plane to go home.

A few hours into the flight, the plane suddenly takes a dive. A frantic flight attendant appears at the front of the aisle, screaming, "The pilot has been growing her hair out to beat the Guinness World Record for Pilot with Longest Hair, but it's in her face and she can't see! Does anyone have seven hundred bobby pins so we can throw her hair into a quick chignon and get this plane back under control?" "I sure do!" I say, and before long, the pilot's hair is up and the plane is back on course. Finally we land, and I think I'm home free, but a couple of IRS agents pull me into an airport interrogation room. "You can't start a sandy lip balm business without checking with us first," they say. "We'll need your complete tax history." "Would all of my receipts since 2003 suffice?" I ask confidently. "Well, yeah," they say. "Actually that'd be fine." Then I walk out of the airport with my empty purse, grateful I carry only the necessities.

Fill your purse with the necessities. You get to define "necessities."

So, now that we've established what you should carry in your bag, here comes the tough part: deciding what kind of bag is best for you. This is a highly personal and often irrational decision (there's no other way to explain my ecstatic purchase of a lime green satin knapsack), but a basic understanding of the four major purse variables can help guide you. The four variables are Size, Material, Shape, and Color.

LET'S START WITH SIZE

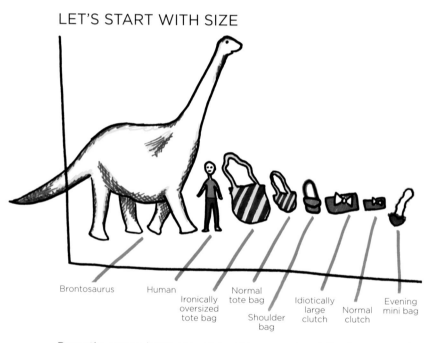

Brontosaurus   Human   Normal tote bag   Evening mini bag

Ironically oversized tote bag   Shoulder bag   Idiotically large clutch   Normal clutch

Recently, purses large enough to hide a murder victim have come into style in a big way. On the other end of the spectrum are evening bags so small, you'd have to make a major effort to fit a lipstick and three dimes inside. So, how to decide what size is best for you? Consider the following questions:

How much stuff are you lugging around?

I'm able to cram my "necessities" into a medium-sized satchel (although I will admit that I've always had a bit of Mary Poppins in me), but if you regularly carry a laptop, or perhaps an anvil, then a larger and sturdier bag may be a better choice. Be careful of going too big, though, as giant totes tend to function less as handbags and more like portals to other worlds where evil ice queens use Turkish delight to lure away your keys and sunglasses.

Where are you lugging it?

I thought it was really cool to carry a gigantic faux-crocodile briefcase to work until I got on a crowded subway train and accidentally hit an angry commuter in the head with it. Another time, I thought it was really cool to use a small clutch as my everyday bag—how trendy and low maintenance!—until its unobtrusive size led me to leave it in a booth at a sandwich shop. It's usually wise to save bags of extreme sizes, small or large, for extreme situations. Take a giant wicker bag to Hawaii. Carry a card deck–sized clutch to the Academy Awards.

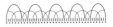

THE MYSTERIOUS PHENOMENON OF THE OVERSIZED CLUTCH

Here's a cautionary limerick about oversized clutches, which have become popular in recent years and should just be called "large bags lacking the convenience of straps":

A chic lady tried clutching a "clutch"

But she found that the weight was too much

Now her back's out of whack

She switched to a small sack

But it's tough to look chic with a crutch

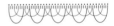

STYLE LESSON #22:

The first person to utter the phrase "happy medium" was probably discussing handbags. It's almost impossible to go wrong with a medium-sized shoulder bag.

What size are you?

As a general rule, very small women should avoid very large bags, and large women should avoid very small bags. Remember Einstein's less-publicized second theory of relativity: *You = HBx5* (Translation: A handbag of about one-fifth your size is always a good choice). Of course, if you want to break this general rule, you have my complete support. No matter your size, it can be fun to carry a statement bag that could double as a hammock, and no woman should ever feel like she's too big to carry that sassy little bejeweled clutch.

MATERIAL

There's not much more to a purse than it's material. Fun details are cool, and cool shapes are fun, but when it comes down to it, a purse is a sack made out of a fabric. To illustrate the vast array of handbag materials and the differences between them, let's take a peek at the Superlatives section of the Handbag High yearbook:

Most Likely to Last Forever: Leather

Most Low Maintenance: Cotton

Most High Maintenance: Suede

Most Likely to Skip School for a Day at the Beach: Wicker

Most Likely to Make You Wish You Could Wear It Rather than Carry It: Cable Knit Cashmere

Most Likely to Make You Go Bankrupt and Look Sort of Cheap Anyway: Snakeskin

Most Likely to be Sort of Cheap but Look Really Expensive: Quilted Leather

Most Likely to Stand You Up for Prom to go on a Hike: Canvas

Most Likely to Get Fake Blood Thrown on You: Mink

Most Likely to Run for Congress in a Random State: Carpet

Most Classy: Silk

Most Casual: Terry cloth

Another material I've fallen in love with recently is clear plastic. Yup. You heard right. To be honest, I wasn't that thrilled when my great-aunt presented me with a see-through handbag that had been sitting in her closet for about thirty years, but I graciously accepted the gift and put it on a shelf in my own closet. Don't get me wrong; I normally love kooky retro accessories, but I'd always felt that clear purses, like sanitary napkin belts, were an idea best left in the history books.

But one fateful day about a week ago, there was an unfortunate granola bar explosion in my usual purse. Its understudy, a bright green flower-print bag, clashed horribly with my outfit, and I was already twenty minutes late. In a panic, I grabbed the clear bag from the closet, dumped the contents of the soiled purse into it, and headed out the door. Here's what I learned that day, and what I remember on the days I carry my clear purse:

A clear purse makes you honest.

No more do I cram my squalor and disorganization behind a neat leather facade and walk around as if I were a tidy, functional adult. Nope. Now, the contents of my purse, and therefore my personality, are right out there, unedited, unashamed.

A clear purse goes with anything.

My love for wild accessories had sort of forced me into dressing around my purses. It's tough to add a giant yellow patent leather handbag to an already colorful outfit and not look like an overly enthusiastic clown. Therefore, I found myself wearing a lot of black. But my clear purse goes with *everything*. Like the Predator, it takes on the appearance of its surroundings, making any outfit plausible.

A clear purse encourages collaboration.

One time, after I got a haircut, I made my way to the front desk and started digging around for the salon gift certificate my boyfriend had given me for Christmas. I had my clear purse up on the counter and was about to launch into my "tee hee how did that receipt from 1998 get in here?" shtick (I do it to fool cashiers into thinking I'm more charming than annoying. It rarely, if ever, works.), when the woman at the desk pointed to the left corner of my clear bag.

"Are you looking for this?" she asked.

I turned the purse around to see what she was talking about, and sure enough, there was my gift certificate, pressed up against the clear plastic. "Yes! Oh my gosh, thank you!"

We both smiled. A messy opaque purse can make for a lonely existence, but a clear purse can turn a potential enemy into an eager teammate.

SHAPE

Modern day handbags come in an infinite variety of silhouettes, from disturbingly small Chihuahua-shaped bags to classic options like satchels and totes; square, circle, and triangle shoulder bags; and so many more.

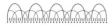

**FASHION RANT:
BACKPACKS**

*Remember the
early '90s when
everyone was wearing
those miniature
backpacks? That was a
sad time for our
country.*

***Here's the deal
with backpacks:***
*Sometimes, you just
need to carry a back-
pack. When you go
backpacking, for exam-
ple. Or if you're in
the fifth grade. In every
other situation, however,
you should seek an
alternative, because
there's no quicker way to
ruin a cute outfit than
to throw a backpack
over the top of it.*

***Healthful
alternatives:***
*Messenger bags,
vintage overnight bags,
extra-large tote
bags, and oversized
slouch bags.*

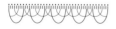

Honestly, the shape of your purse is totally up to you. If you play the tri-angle professionally, you might want to avoid a circular bag, but other than that, choose whatever shape appeals to you, and read on to see what the stars say about your choice.

Horoscopes Based on Your Preferred Bag Shape

➤ **MOON-SHAPED SATCHEL:** Today will be an excellent day for you if you can avoid that swarm of killer bees.

➤ **SLOUCHY TRIANGLE SHOULDER BAG:** There's never been a better time to pluck your eyebrows.

➤ **SQUARE TOTE:** Today you will be tempted by a tall, dark, handsome man and a deceptively edible-smelling vanilla body wash. Resist both.

➤ **RECTANGLE CLUTCH:** Eating cookies for breakfast isn't the best idea, but a girl's gotta do what a girl's gotta do.

➤ **CIRCULAR WRISTLET:** If it sounds like the pigeons are talking to you, it's because they are.

COLOR

The one purse color that matches everything is black. If you were or still are one of those kids who went to school all cocky in the second grade with your newfound knowledge that black technically is not a color, but rather the absence of color, I really don't care. The fact is, if you want a bag that will look truly good with every single outfit, black is the color for you. The downside? It's a little boring.

Moving on to neutrals that match almost everything, we have brown, tan, cream, and cranberry. Yes, cranberry. Name one color that doesn't look good next to cranberry. You can't? Yeah, that's what I thought. These col-ors are perfect for work, because they're a little more interesting than black but still go with every outfit and look professional.

In the no-man's-land between neutrals and bright colors live the metal-lics. Silver, gold, or bronze purses are super cute and look great with almost any outfit. They're not as adaptable as the true neutrals, since they're not the best choice for more conservative work environments, but they're surprisingly versatile.

Last but not least, we have the "pop of color" purses. This group encompasses the crazy bright colors—pumpkin orange, fire-engine red, lime green, royal blue, canary yellow—that instantly make an outfit exciting and fresh. They're hard to pull off as everyday bags, unless you wear all black all the time and can handle the constant color popping, but they're fantastic options to own when you need a lift (emotionally or fashionably speaking). Feeling brave? Wear your pop of color purse with a pop of color outfit. See the color wheel below for an illustration of purse color concepts. The circles radiate outward from the most versatile color option (black) to less versatile, more fun options.

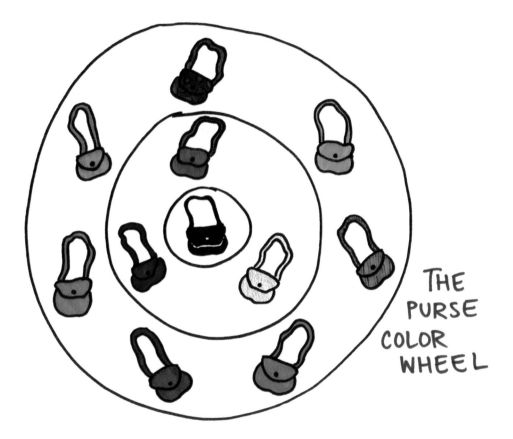

THE
PURSE
COLOR
WHEEL

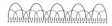
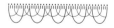
Speaking of Colors, Should You Match Your Purse to Your Shoes? Or Your Shoes to Your Purse? Aaaahhh, I'm So Confused!

This area of fashion formulae is totally confusing, because in the span of about five years, shoe and purse matching went from a fashion MUST DO to a humiliating fashion GOD NO. I reside pretty strongly in the anti-matching camp, but here's my take on the situation: if your purse and shoes both happen to be, like, black, then don't worry about it. If, however, you're under eighty-five and are rocking a coordinated electric blue crocodile skin tote and loafer combo, you might want to reconsider. Unless you're making an ironic postmodern so-bad-it's-good statement, which could be sort of awesome. Do you see why I say there are no fashion rules anymore?

SHOPPING FOR PURSES

In my humble opinion, shopping for purses is a certifiable Fun Fest. You don't have to try anything on, every item fits perfectly, and you can experiment with crazy styles without risking your self-worth. Deciding how much to spend and where to shop for your new handbag(s) depends on how you would (honestly) answer the following question:

Are you a purse slut?

If you go through multiple purses a week, never satisfied, constantly bored, always craving excitement, adventure, and change, then you are a purse slut and should stick to less expensive purses. Shop at discount retailers, sale racks, thrift stores, and department stores for funky bags to feed your cravings, but make sure to add a few fairly basic options to your purse wardrobe.

STYLE LESSON #23:

It's never good, twenty minutes before an important job interview, to be frantically debating between the neon yellow striped satchel and the red and green clutch shaped like a watermelon. Always have a basic, versatile handbag option on standby.

If you're more the "find a nice purse and settle down type," it makes sense to spend some money—a shocking amount of money, even—on a truly quality purse, because with a little care, you could use it literally every day for the next fifty years.

Personally, my fear of commitment has kept me from taking the luxury purse plunge (yep, I'm a purse slut), but I clearly remember the first time one of my friends dropped some major dollars on a designer bag. I was a sophomore in college when it happened. My friend Kathy announced that she had just purchased a Marc Jacobs handbag for the price of $1,300. Up until then, my $50 splurges at TJ Maxx had made me the "big spender" of our group, so this was a pretty huge deal.

After Kathy brought her purchase home, she didn't take it out of the bag for hours. She called me that night and talked about it like it was a wild animal that had no business in her room. "It's just sitting there in the corner! I'm scared to touch it!"

It took me a while to adjust to this new paradigm. Whenever I rode in my boyfriend's car, I couldn't help but remember that Kathy's wallet was being carried around in a leather sack worth a hundred bucks more than the 1987 Honda Accord carrying ME around. The realization left me dumbfounded. All wallets should be so lucky.

When to Get a New Bag

A lot of women in past generations had a different purse (or purses) for each season—maybe a straw bag for summer, a brown suede bag for fall/winter, and a cotton tote for spring. This is a great way to prolong the lives of your purses and to get a fresh look for each season. But if you're more the type to stick with one bag until it falls apart, try to draw the line when your purse is literally falling apart. I once had a purple bag that I loved more than my family, but by the end of its run, it was crumbling, the strap was broken (I had to cradle it like an infant, but I didn't mind), and strange bonelike rods were protruding from the bottom. If a good friend hadn't acted in the nick of time by throwing it away and presenting me with a gorgeous replacement, I would have swathed that sad, bony piece of leather in a hand-knit baby blanket and carried it to this day. God, I miss that purse. What was I talking about again?

Oh yes, reasons to change your bag. Another excellent impetus for a bag change is if you are upset or bored with your life. I've discussed how a woman's bag is really a metaphor for her life, so changing your purse can be a surprisingly powerful statement. Get yourself a new bag to jump-start a big life change, or reward yourself for an event that's already happened.

THE TAO OF THE HANDBAG

Just in case you haven't been paying attention at all, allow me to recap: handbags are much more significant than most people give them credit for. A purse can be an extension of your home, a single girl's baby, a security blanket when walking into a party full of good-looking people, a weapon when walking home alone, a way to smuggle sodas and sushi platters into the movie theater, the perfect addition to an amazing outfit, or the one thing that makes a boring outfit amazing. The list goes on and on and on.

Take your handbags seriously, but not too seriously. Have fun with colors, shapes, and sizes, and build up a personal purse supply that can cure even the dreariest bouts of "Gaaahhh, I hate all my clothes!" Stock your bags with stuff that makes you happy, and maybe some practical things too, like lip balm with sand in it. Hey, you never know.

SEVEN

"This Coat Isn't Waterproof"

AND OTHER CAUTIONARY TALES AND TIPS ON OUTERWEAR

MY GRANDMA ALWAYS USED TO SAY, "A girl's gotta have a good coat!" Well, actually she didn't. More often, she said things like, "Don't tell your mother I let you ride to the store in the car trunk," but I wish she would have told me to have a good coat, because that would have been true and applicable and much less likely to cause personal injury or death.

Listen to your grandmother (unless she tells you to get in the trunk): a girl's gotta have a good coat!

I'm a staunch believer that when it comes to outerwear, quality counts. I love trendy, inexpensive clothes as much as the next girl, but I've never, ever regretted laying down the extra Benjamins for a well-made coat, for two reasons. First of all, coats keep you warm, and warm = alive. Who knows, if Luke Skywalker had invested in quality outerwear, maybe Han Solo wouldn't have had to stick him in a disemboweled tauntaun. Secondly, and perhaps more importantly, an unsightly coat can, in an instant, render all your other fashion efforts irrelevant. How many times have you spent hours planning the perfect outfit for an important event, and then, at the first sign of rain or cold, had to cover it all up with a tatty, unflattering jacket? No matter how stylish you are underneath, the world will only see a tragic case of outerwear.

Case in point: once, I had to go to court to dispute a speeding ticket. I was seventeen and had been caught careening down my small town's main street at 73 miles per hour, on my way to turn in an important history paper that, in retrospect, was not important at all. After sobbing to the state trooper about the vital importance of said history paper, I was issued a citation for $250. I felt an immediate rush of panic at the thought of telling my dad, combined with excitement at the chance to wear a dramatically demure outfit to court and plead my innocence.

I spent weeks planning a foolproof outfit and defense. I would wear a cream skirt with flower embroidery, a black shirt with pearl buttons and a rounded collar, black tights, ballet flats, a red vintage scarf, and round sunglasses. I would say if society wanted to persecute me for striving to be a good student, then I would dutifully pay the price; but I would forever lament the injustice of a legal system that so callously ignored a citizen's right to life, liberty, and the 73-miles-per-hour pursuit of an A on an essay about the industrial revolution.

The day of my court appearance, everything went according to plan: my outfit looked great, and my note cards were in order. When I walked out the door, I felt a raindrop, so I ran back inside and grabbed a random coat from the laundry room. This random coat happened to be my mom's dilapidated fleece pullover, but I didn't think much of it as I slipped it on and headed to the courthouse.

When I arrived, I strutted through the big doors and down the hall to my assigned courtroom. I whipped off my glamorous shades and faced a huge room packed with traffic offenders and nonviolent felons. People were glaring and the judge's bench was much more imposing than I'd anticipated and the whole thing was decidedly unglamorous.

The judge came in and the clerk started calling names for rapid-fire public pleas. I was hyperventilating. About fifteen minutes in, they called my name. I stood up on wobbly legs and they asked me for my plea. I opened my mouth to speak, but suddenly all I could think was "Oh my God, I'm wearing a fleece covered in dog hair."

"Guilty," I said.

STYLE LESSON #25:

Everyone judges a book by its cover; make sure your cover isn't made of ratty fleece.

You can prepare yourself for every style and weather situation by building an outerwear wardrobe that includes the following pieces:

➤ **A waterproof jacket**

➤ **A black wool peacoat**

➤ **A coat warm enough to keep you alive** through the next ice age (or a winter weekend in Chicago)

➤ **A unique coat** in the perfect color that puts all eyes on you

NOTE: *To those who live in perpetually warm climates and refuse to make friends farther from the equator: Yes, you are allowed to skip this chapter. Take the money you're saving and spend it on sunscreen and lottery tickets. See ya in about ten pages.*

A WATERPROOF JACKET

"Waterproof," to my father, means the wearer can experience a monsoon, in a sinking boat, and come home to dinner later saying, "It rained? Really? I didn't notice." Not an ounce of moisture should be able to penetrate a jacket that makes the highfalutin claim to be waterproof.

"Waterproof," to me, means not suede.

This difference of opinion came to a head when I went to outdoor school in the sixth grade. I'd gotten one of those awesome raincoats from Gap that folds up into a little matching bag, and I was so excited to show my classmates my fashion prowess.

My dad saw the coat the night before my departure. I was carefully folding it and placing it in my suitcase when I heard, "*What is that?*"

Too late to hide it, I told the truth. "My new coat," I said. "Why?"

He took the coat out of my hands and squinted at the seams. He turned it inside out and ran his fingers along the fabric, frowning. "This coat isn't waterproof," he sighed.

"I'm sure it's fine," I stammered. "I'm, I'm sure it won't rain while I'm there, and if it does, I'm sure it will be fine."

"No, no, no," he muttered, as he got up and carried the coat to his office. "I'll fix it for you." I followed him, pleading with him to just let his daughter get rained on, for once, but he wasn't listening. He laid the coat out on his desk and rifled through a drawer. "Here it is." He pulled out a silver tube, took off the cap, and started squirting white goo onto the seams of my precious new coat.

"What is that?" I asked in horror.

"Sealant," he said. "Keeps the water out."

The first day at outdoor school, there was a rainstorm. The teachers had a stack of garbage bags for the kids without coats. I looked at my raincoat, smeared with bathroom sealant that was flaking off like dried skin, and stuffed it back in my suitcase. Then I got in line for a garbage bag.

To avoid wearing a garbage bag, take this handy quiz to figure out what style of waterproof coat is for you, and then find your corresponding ideal outerwear on the following pages.

Your idea of a perfect weekend is:

a. **A strenuous hike in the mountains with your dog.**

b. **Leaving the love of your life on an airport tarmac to fly to Lisbon with your husband to join the Nazi-resistance movement.**

If you answered "A strenuous hike in the mountains with your dog":

You might enjoy a Sporty, Hardcore Waterproof Jacket!

FEATURES:

➤ **Actually, seriously, truly waterproof.** As in, my dad would have no urge to squirt sealant on the seams.

➤ **Lots of bells and whistles**—armpit zippers, nylon cords, mesh lining, built-in canteens.

➤ **Usually more functional than fashionable,** but can easily be worked into an outdoorsy wardrobe and, with a little creativity, worn with trendier pieces.

WEAR IT WITH:

➤ **Distressed jeans**

➤ **Black yoga pants**

➤ **Workout gear**

➤ **Denim skirts and knit leggings**

➤ **Jersey dresses**

WHERE TO BUY:

➤ **Outdoors retailers** (including catalogs and online)

➤ **Sportswear stores**

➤ **Outlet malls**

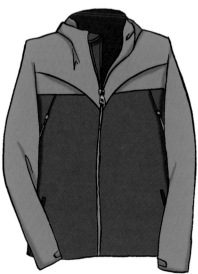

If you enjoy dramatic good-byes at the Casablanca airport:

A Classic Trench Coat may be the right choice for you!

FEATURES:

➤ **The true classic trench** is tan canvas or nylon, belted, and long (to the ankle).

➤ **Newer incarnations can be brightly colored,** cropped, hooded, cotton, wool, patterned, and feature different lengths of sleeves and belts. Somehow, even a hot-pink trench (I have one) looks classic and refined.

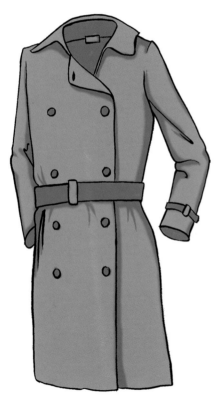

➤ **Some versions are more waterproof than others,** but most will keep you dry, at least for a while.

➤ **This style of coat,** along with the black wool peacoat, will never, ever go out of style. Buy one to enjoy and to pass down to your daughter, granddaughter, and great-granddaughter ten times removed. Heck, have yourself cryogenically frozen with your trench coat, then wake up and wear it in five hundred years: you'll be showered with compliments on your "fresh and current" style.

WEAR IT WITH:

➤ **Jeans**

➤ **Trousers**

➤ **Fun hosiery**

➤ **Wrap dresses**

➤ **Printed skirts**

WHERE TO BUY:

➤ **Department stores**

➤ **High-end designer boutiques**

➤ **Vintage stores** (see for yourself that these things last for hundreds of years)

THE PERFECT PEACOAT

The next style of coat I recommend is the black wool peacoat. Take this handy quiz to determine if you need one yourself.

So, how much do you love peacoats?

a. OMG. I loooooove peacoats!

b. I love peacoats with the fire of a thousand suns.

c. I would totally marry a peacoat if my friends wouldn't judge me.

STYLE LESSON #26:

Seriously, everyone needs a black wool peacoat.

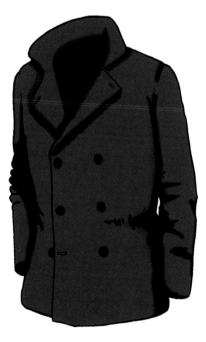

Black wool peacoats look good with everything, from gray sweats (well, nothing looks good with gray sweats, but a black wool peacoat looks better than most things) to jeans to party dresses to military uniforms. They look good on everyone, and they are always in style.

I'm not kidding when I say everyone needs one. Sure, they might not be the most exciting purchase, but they are a flattering, versatile basic you'll end up wearing all the time, and you'll look and feel chic.

So, say I've convinced you to get a peacoat (no, really, I want to hear you say it). Now it's time to confront that age-old question—single- or double-breasted?

The Single-Breasted vs. Double-Breasted Debate: A Play in One Act

PEACOAT MODERATOR: First of all, I'd like to thank you both for joining us.

SINGLE-BREASTED: Glad to be here.

DOUBLE-BREASTED: Double glad to be here.

MODERATOR: I'll start with you, Single-Breasted. Why are you the best choice?

SINGLE-BREASTED: Goodness, where to begin? I'm sleek, modern, and slimming. I don't add bulk, so I'm great for women with larger busts or broad shoulders.

MODERATOR: And you, Double-Breasted?

DOUBLE-BREASTED: Listen, I think there's absolutely no question that I'm the classic choice. Sailors, models, and hipsters have worn me for generations. I'm smart and retro cool.

MODERATOR: Double-Breasted, would you agree with the assertion that Single-Breasted is a better choice for women with larger busts or broad shoulders?

DOUBLE-BREASTED: Well, yeah. But those women can definitely wear me too. If they keep the bottoms of their outfits slim and streamlined, they'll look great.

SINGLE-BREASTED: Exactly.

MODERATOR: Well, this isn't really a debate at all.

WHERE TO BUY:

➤ **Department stores**

➤ **Military surplus stores**

➤ **Vintage shops**

➤ **Estate sales**

A COAT WARM ENOUGH TO KEEP YOU ALIVE THROUGH THE NEXT ICE AGE (OR A WINTER WEEKEND IN CHICAGO)

To determine which type of warm coat is best for you, please consult the Regional Outerwear Reference Map below:

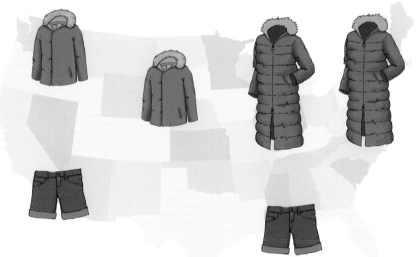

As a longtime resident of the "pretty cold" region, I once made the mistake of complaining to a friend about a slight chill in the air. This was a mistake because (1) it really wasn't that cold outside, and (2) my friend had gone to college in Chicago.

"Do you want to hear what I wore every morning in the winter in Chicago just to walk to the damn bus stop?" she demanded, and I said yes.

"First, I put on some leggings and an undershirt. Then thermal underwear over that. Then I put on some flannel pants. Then a turtleneck. And a down vest. Leg warmers. Arm warmers. A ski mask . . . "

I lost the next three minutes of my life to a tireless and detailed description of her Chicago survival-dressing ritual. I started to laugh when I imagined her waddling around in seven layers of pants, but she shot me a glare so icy, I remained stone-faced even when she described stuffing a throw pillow under her shirt for extra warmth.

" . . . And then I put on earmuffs. And one of those Russian fur hats. And gloves. And mittens. And the sheepskin rug from my living room. And my quilted down jacket. And then I walked to the bus stop and I was still cold."

"Jesus," I whispered.

"Yeah," she said.

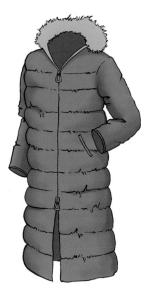

STYLE LESSON #27:

If you live, have lived, or ever plan to live north of the Mason-Dixon Line, you might want to consider one of those giant quilted jackets that look like a queen-size down comforter with sleeves.

FEATURES:

➤ **This coat may or may not** have begun its life as a down comforter, but that's OK, because it will keep you alive.

WEAR IT WITH:

➤ **Doesn't really matter,** because you're wearing a blanket.

➤ **Throw pillows.**

WHERE TO BUY:

➤ **Outerwear and sportswear stores**

➤ **Department stores** in colder climates

➤ **The cute little boutique** at Everest's base camp

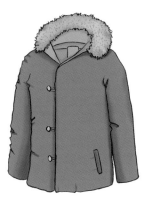

If you live in the "cold" region and don't want to wear a floor-length blanket coat, try a hooded parka.

A hooded parka won't provide as much warmth as a down comforter coat, but it will keep you relatively toasty and dry without making you look like a queen size bed.

FEATURES:

➤ **Different versions** made from different fabrics, but quilted down is the most common.

➤ **Fun details:** bright colors, different lengths, buttons, zippers, toggles, and faux fur–lined hoods.

➤ **Hooded parkas,** especially colorful quilted ones, look young and sporty. They can add a funky twist to more conservative outfits, but be careful of pairing them with a miniskirt and sneakers, because you'll look like you're twelve.

WEAR IT WITH:

➤ **Skirts, thick tights, and boots**

➤ **Wool pants**

➤ **Jeans** (optional: six layers of pants underneath)

WHERE TO BUY:

➤ **Department stores**

➤ **Outdoors stores**

➤ **Discount retailers and Web sites**

NOTE: *If you live in a cold region but can't see yourself ever donning a quilted coat or a hooded parka, invest in a wide-collared, button-down cream or camel wool coat. You might have to stuff a throw pillow underneath to ensure you'll be warm enough, but even so, a classic wool coat always looks chic.*

A UNIQUE COAT IN THE PERFECT COLOR THAT PUTS ALL EYES ON YOU (PREFERABLY WITH AN INTRIGUING BACKSTORY, LIKE "THERE WAS ONLY ONE LEFT AND IT WAS IN MY SIZE!" OR "THIS OLD THING? I FOUND IT AT A LITTLE VINTAGE SHOP IN TEXAS FOR TWENTY BUCKS!")

This one is pretty self-explanatory, right? It's important to have a fun, flattering, showstopping coat that makes you feel fantastic. This coat is

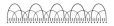

SHOULD MY COAT BE A SIZE BIGGER TO ACCOMMODATE LAYERS?

I've gone with this approach in the past, only to be disappointed by a permanently baggy coat. If you live north of the Mason-Dixon Line, then do what you must, but generally I think it's better to get a coat that fits you properly, and then wear quality thinner layers underneath—cashmere sweaters (bought on sale, of course!), for example.

DOES MY COAT HAVE TO BE THE SAME LENGTH AS MY SKIRT OR DRESS, OR DID THAT RULE BECOME OBSOLETE IN, LIKE, 1873?

That rule pretty much became obsolete in 1873. I think it's so fun—and fashionable—to play with layers and proportions in your outerwear. The hem of a colorful dress peeking out below a trench coat looks very modern. Try out different combinations and see what you like!

continues »

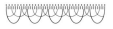

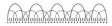

continued »

CROPPED COATS MAKE ME LOOK LIKE A MINI-FRIDGE. WHAT SHOULD I DO?

Try a coat that hits at your hips or lower. And definitely don't wear children's artwork on your chest.

I'M REALLY SORRY, BUT I THINK BLACK WOOL PEACOATS ARE SORT OF BORING. IS THERE A WAY TO SPICE THEM UP?

I'll give you FIVE ways:

*1.
Wear a colorful vintage scarf around your neck.*

*2.
Choose a peacoat with a pretty silk lining, or have a tailor put one in for you.*

*3.
Pin a fabric corsage to your lapel.*

*4.
Replace the plain buttons with gaudy gold ones (or whatever you please).*

*5.
Wear a rainbow sequin singlet underneath.*

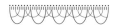

special. You should be able to walk down a crowded street in this coat and not see another one like it for MILES. If you don't own a coat like this yet, here are some ideas.

➤ **Retro red swing jacket:** Wear this eye-catching piece on a date or to a job interview—you're sure to be remembered.

➤ **Black-and-white herringbone cape:** Gorgeous at a ladies' lunch or independent film festival, a cape makes any outfit look special.

➤ **Neon green '80s nylon jacket:** Wear it to a concert, roller skating, or for a Saturday stroll in the park.

➤ **Cropped leather bomber in any color:** Throw your bomber jacket over a simple tee and jeans for a day of shopping, or a sweet frilly dress for a summer night out.

➤ **Tie-dyed denim jacket:** Try a bohemian denim jacket with a classic black sweater dress for Sunday coffee with friends.

➤ **Long felt coat with faux fur cuffs and collar:** Perfect for winter weddings or funerals. Also, the office Christmas party.

➤ **Plaid belted overcoat:** Classic menswear pieces look amazing with skirts, subtly textured tights, and high-heeled Mary Janes.

Keep your eyes open at the mall, flea markets, vintage shops, boutiques, and your grandma's closet, but don't force this purchase. Like love, you can't hurry your perfect coat: when you see it, you'll just know. For my friend Catherine, it's a bright yellow single-breasted peacoat. For my mom, it's a felt maroon princess coat from Gap that miraculously goes with everything she owns. In high school, my best friend Rachel had a fuzzy orange coat that sparked rumors she had poached and skinned an orangutan (it was acrylic), but she loved that coat with a burning passion. The stares weren't just worth it—they were the point.

EIGHT

The Little Touches:

HOW TO MAKE AN ENTRANCE WITH JEWELRY, SCARVES, HATS, BELTS, AND SUNGLASSES

ACCESSORIES ARE ARGUABLY THE MOST IMPORTANT ASPECT of your wardrobe. Sure, clothes can save you from indecent exposure charges, but with the right accessories, you can look good even while being booked into prison. In this chapter, I cover the bitter little group of accessories left over once shoes and bags are given their own chapters, specifically: jewelry, scarves, hats, belts, and sunglasses.

JEWELRY

In the past ten years or so, many previously inflexible fashion rules have gone out the window. "No white shoes after Labor Day," "Match your purse to your shoes," and "Don't wear a shirt as a dress, but if you do, please wear underwear," are now archaic remnants of the stuffy style of the past.

My favorite dead style rule goes something like this: "Your earrings should match your necklace, which should match your bracelet, which should match your outfit. Ideally, you should also change your jewelry at every meal to match the colors of your shepherd's pie or seafood linguine."

My mom was always a die-hard jewelry matcher. Many mornings I would catch her staring in the mirror above her jewelry box, clutching a fistful of earrings, frozen in panic. "What's wrong?" I'd ask, and she'd explain how she really, really wanted to wear her new blue earrings, but she couldn't because there wasn't any blue in the floral pattern of her blouse.

"Why don't you just wear them anyway?"

She'd glare at me, one eyebrow raised, as if I had just suggested that she become a communist.

"I *can't*," she'd sigh, and then she would do one of two things: slowly and dejectedly put back the blue earrings, or get out the magnifying glass she kept in her dresser and scour the minuscule floral print on her shirt for the slightest hint of blue to justify her earring urges.

STYLE LESSON #28:

Compulsive jewelry matching can drive a woman insane. Wear jewelry you love with clothing you love: it's that simple.

Luckily for me, sometime in the late '90s, the Fundamentalist Church of the Matchy-Matchy died, and these days, anything goes, especially when it comes to jewelry. Want to wear blue earrings with an orange shirt? Go for it! Silver necklace with pearl earrings with gold bracelet? More power to you!

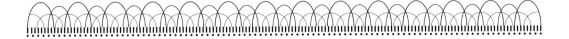

Six Types of Jewelry You Should Never, Ever, Under Any Circumstances, Get Rid of, Because if You Do, You Will Live a Life of Sadness and Regret

CUFF OR BANGLE BRACELETS
Small, medium, or large, these pretty pieces are a great finishing touch to your outfit.

SIMPLE GOLD OR SILVER CHAINS
Classic, flattering, and versatile. I challenge you to make a chain necklace look anything but elegant.

JEWELED BROOCH
Yes, brooches can come off as a bit septuagenarian, but balance them with dazzling youth and/or funky clothing you'll be fine.

LARGE COCKTAIL RINGS
Always, always in style.

PEARLS
I once wore my triple-strand pearl necklace to conduct an interview in a chicken coop. The interview went really well, which leads me to conclude that pearls are appropriate and beneficial to every possible life situation.

ANYTHING WITH A FAMILY HISTORY
Accessories, and especially jewelry, are a really special way for generations of women to relate to and honor each other. My great-grandma left me four inexpensive Timex watches that don't tell time anymore, but sometimes I'll stack them all on my wrist and be four times as late as I normally am, which is OK, because they make me think of her. All my friends have favorite memories of playing with their moms' jewelry or trying on hats (or wigs) with their great-aunts.

And a Few Pieces of Jewelry Maybe You Should Get Rid of:

TOE RINGS
Like toe socks, these are best left in the goodie bags of middle school birthday parties.

EARRINGS SHAPED LIKE MINIATURE SOUVENIRS
I still own a pair of purple-haired troll doll earings from the early '90s, and they are just as terrifying as they sound.

BOLO TIES
It takes a truckload of irony to pull this look off, and truck rentals ain't cheap.

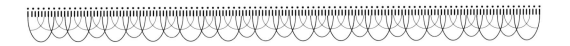

STYLE LESSON #29:

Even if a piece of your grandma's jewelry is absolutely, totally not your style, do me a favor and tuck it away somewhere. You'll be very glad you did.

Some general tips for adorning yourself to the fullest:

1. **Department store jewelry can be overpriced** and unoriginal. Widen your jewelry shopping scope and dig up great finds at garage and estate sales, thrift stores, vintage boutiques, antique malls, and street markets. The jewelry you'll find at these places is inexpensive (often no more than $10), unique, and includes bragging rights ("Oh, this gorgeous, one-of-a-kind pendant? I found it at a random garage sale for fifty cents!")

2. **Raid your mother's or grandmother's closet** for groovy retro pieces that yearn to escape the confines of the "matching set."

3. **Layer necklaces of various lengths, colors, and styles** to add interest to any outfit. Same goes for bracelets.

4. **Try pairing big, bold costume jewelry** with jeans and a T-shirt and tell me you're not the coolest girl in the room.

5. **Don't pile approximately thirty black rubber bracelet**s on each arm in an effort to look cool and edgy only to find out later that said bracelets are widely used to symbolize sexual experience. Not that I did this in the seventh grade.

As with shoes and handbags, jewelry gives us a great opportunity to have fun with fashion. Even if you normally wear very classic, simple clothing, there's no reason you can't be a jewelry trendsetter. Experiment with different pieces and combinations to create a look that's all your own. Remember, all it takes is one eye-popping necklace to go from "Sort of Boring Girl" to "Awesome Eye-Popping Necklace Girl."

HATS

Back in the day, an outfit wasn't an outfit until it was topped off with a beautiful hat. Today we live in a sad, dark, relatively hatless world. I strongly believe that more women should take advantage of these fun, flattering, and useful accessories, because hats look good on almost everyone, and more importantly, they can give the illusion that you put some effort into your outfit. Put on a hat, even if only to cover up an epically bad hair day, and suddenly you're "put together."

The Hat Survey

BEANIE

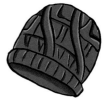

Wear it to . . . the mall, the skate park, movie night, running errands, lunch dates.

Wear it with . . . casual jeans and a tank top, or throw on a slouchy beanie with a dress and opaque tights—so sexy!

Get one for free if . . . you steal it from an injured skateboarder.

WIDE-BRIMMED SUN HAT

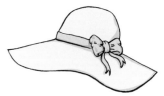

Wear it to . . . the beach, the pool, the Kentucky Derby.

Wear it with . . . a swimsuit, sarong, or sundress.

Get one for free if . . . you hit the beach on a windy day (finders keepers!).

FEDORA

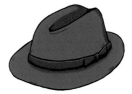

Wear it to . . . outdoor lunches, walks around the city, organized crime meetings.

Wear it with . . . jeans, dresses, or cutoffs and a tank top in the summertime.

Get one for free if . . . you assassinate a mob boss.

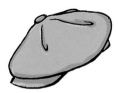

NEWSBOY CAP

Wear it to . . . weekend getaways, tooling around town, grocery shopping.

Wear it with . . . a simple white T-shirt and slouchy trousers.

Get one for free if . . . you sell papers on Chicago street corners circa 1935.

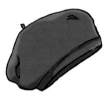

BERET

Wear it to . . . art school to intimidate your classmates, Paris to piss off the locals.

Wear it with . . . striped shirts, breezy dresses, baguettes.

Get one for free if . . . you join the army special forces (offer redeemable for green beret only).

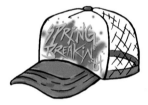

TRUCKER HAT

Wear it to . . . frat parties, long-haul transport runs of goods.

Wear it with . . . sports jerseys, bikinis, white T-shirts (wet).

Get one for free if . . . you flash your breasts for the cameras while on spring break.

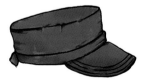

FIDEL CASTRO CAP

Wear it to . . . hipster bars, college classes, the revolution.

Wear it with . . . skinny jeans, vintage T-shirts, Converse.

Get one for free if . . . you stage a political coup.

SOMBRERO

Wear it to . . . traditional Mexican celebrations.

Wear it with . . . umm, pride?

Get one for free if . . . you have your birthday celebration at a festive Mexican restaurant.

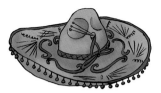

SCARVES

Pretty much everyone agrees French women always look chic. So what's their big secret? Do you really want to know?

Scarves.

Seriously, look closely at any photo of a stunning French woman, and you'll see she's wearing her Michigan State sweats, an old T-shirt from one of those supermarket three-packs, and a blindingly chic scarf.

STYLE LESSON #30:

The only difference between you and a stylish French woman is that she has a gorgeous scarf around her neck.

Scarves and hats are very similar in that they take very little effort—extend arm, grab scarf and/or hat, put it on—but have the power to upgrade or transform a whole look. No matter your hurry or mood, there's no excuse not to throw on a colorful scarf or a cool-looking hat (or both).

To make things even easier, there is really no such thing as a bad scarf, so the details are up to you. Wide scarves, skinny scarves, warm scarves, printed scarves, solid scarves, sequined scarves, cheap scarves, expensive scarves—I love and own them all. You could make one designer silk scarf your signature look or wear a different scarf every day. Either way, you'll look amazing.

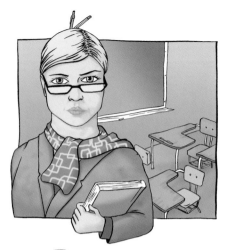

How to Wear a Scarf without Looking Like an English Teacher

One question that comes up a lot is how to wear a square silk scarf without looking like a stern English teacher.

Here are a few ways to wear your silk scarf that won't cause passersby to avert their eyes in hopes of avoiding a lecture on appropriate comma usage:

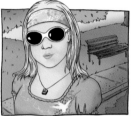

1. THE SCARF-AS-HEADBAND

You can vary the level of subtlety depending on how wide you fold the scarf (just fold it to the desired size and tie it under your hair). It can either be a nice little shot of color holding your hair back, or you can create a really wide headband, tease your hair up eight inches, and wear huge sunglasses for a more dramatic '60s effect.

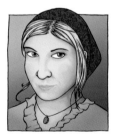

2. FRENCH PEASANT CHIC

Folding your scarf into a triangle and tying it around your head may have dusty connotations (as in actually dusting), but as long as it's a cute scarf and you're not wearing ratty sweatpants and carrying a duster, I swear this look can work.

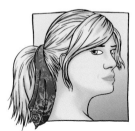

3. THE PERFECT PONYTAIL

Tie your scarf around a ponytail or wrap it around a bun for a simple, preppy look. Have fun playing with different colors against your hair.

4. THE PIRATE/HOLLYWOOD STARLET

Let your hair down and fold the scarf into a triangle, then tie it straight across your forehead, knotting it in the back. Add gold teeth and goatee for a pirate costume, or huge aviators, trendy peace sign, and coked-out stare for a perfect impression of a celebrity beach bunny. Or maybe not.

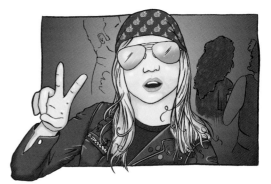

Other options include threading your scarf through your belt loops, tying it to your handbag, or wearing it under a blazer like a tie. Do some experimenting and have fun with it, but leave your teacher's edition of *The Great Gatsby* at home, just to be safe.

SUNGLASSES

There are two schools of thought when it comes to shopping for sunglasses, and if these schools of thought were literally schools, they would be rivals, and the annual homecoming game would be extremely tense.

The first school, the Disposers (ooh, intimidating!), believe sunglasses get broken all the time (true) and should therefore be viewed as disposable and unsentimental. Sit down in your car and hear that familiar crunch? Oh well! People with this attitude tend to have stockpiles of $5 sunglasses stashed in their homes, cars, offices, and body cavities.

On the opposite end of the spectrum are the Investors. These people spend a chunk of change on quality sunglasses and quality cases to protect them. Their sunglasses last for years, thanks to good care and protection, but in the event of breakage, Investors are often emotionally distraught and unprepared. In addition, if Investors are not careful to choose timeless styles, they will still be wearing Maui Jims in 2050.

Luckily, there are many options available for both schools. Disposers now enjoy a huge selection of cheap, cute sunglasses at affordable retailers and discount stores, while Investors can find expensive, beautiful options at any number of department stores and boutiques. Both teams are well served by online auction sites as well.

I straddle the line by buying formerly expensive designer sunglasses at discount stores or during major sales. This strategy fulfills my fashionista urge to keep a gaudy designer name close to my temple, and my responsible urge to keep a few dollars in my wallet. An acquaintance once tried to convince me that buying knockoffs was the way to go, but as soon as I saw her "Guchi" frames, I knew it wasn't for me.

How to Choose the Best Sunglasses for Your Face

SIZE

At the risk of sounding like a spam e-mail subject line, bigger really is better when it comes to sunglasses. You know how low-budget horror movie productions will put a human in a monster suit next to a miniaturized skyline, and all of a sudden the monster looks huge and scary and menacing? Small sunglasses have a similar effect on your head. Even though you possess a nice, normal-sized cranium, small sunglasses will make it look huge and scary and menacing. I'm sorry. It's true.

A pair of oversized sunglasses is the rare fashion item that makes you look chic *and* hides imperfections (unlike, say, a satin mini dress). Have a bad hangover? A zit on your cheek? Lose an eye playing racquetball? Slip on a pair of big, dark sunglasses, and the world will never know.

SHAPE

I've always enjoyed the rule of opposites: whatever the shape of your face, choose frames that are the opposite shape. If your face is more circular, try square frames; if you're more of a square (no offense), go for rounder frames. And remember, whatever shape you go for, go big.

Extra Tips for Staring into the Sun in Style

➤ **Sunglasses are a good way** to take a fashion risk without, well, risking much. Try colorful, embellished, mirrored, seriously oversized, or even heart-shaped frames (or all of the above!). Thrift stores have tons of fun sunglasses abandoned by cowardly owners—adopt them for a couple of bucks and stand out in a crowd.

➤ **Aviators and Jackie O. frames** look good on everyone.

➤ **Wear sunglasses at night** only if you're performing karaoke to "I Wear My Sunglasses at Night" and want to make a point.

BELTS

I have a complex relationship with belts. As someone with a slightly rotund gut, I hear the belt solution a lot. "Just throw on a belt," chirp the fashion advice columnists. "Voila! Instant hourglass figure!"

But here's the thing: That's a giant lie. See, my body shape is eerily similar to a frog's.

Fashion magazines would advise a frog to wrap a belt around its waist, the widest part of its body. Fashion magazines claim this frog would subsequently enjoy an hourglass figure. Apparently, fashion magazines have never actually tested this theory (see illustration).

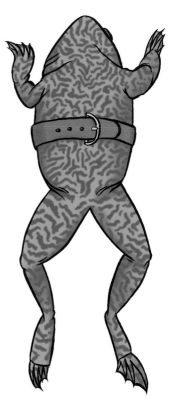

STYLE LESSON #31:

Don't put a belt on a frog.

Now, don't get me wrong, frog-shaped readers can still enjoy fulfilling, belted lives. Just because the instant hourglass figure thing is a cruel urban legend doesn't mean you can't find a flattering belt placement on your body. Try above your waist, lower on your hips (basically anywhere but your widest part), or get creative—put a cute belt through your belt loops and use it to hold your pants up.

Those lucky gals whose shapes are more hourglass than amphibious have a bit more freedom to explore their belting desires. Cinching an already-defined waist with a belt looks quite fetching, and if your waist is the smallest part of your torso, it's quite slimming too.

Belt it out!

➤ **As I discussed in the jewelry section,** the matchy-matchy look is passé. There's no need to match your belt to your shoes to your bag—experiment with different color and texture combinations to liven up your look.

- **The next time you accidentally walk into** a fabulous but shockingly overpriced boutique, check out the belt rack—belts are almost always under $50.

- **Look for random giant belt buckles** everywhere from garage sales to department stores. Wear with flared jeans and a tight black tank top, or over a too-pretty dress to toughen it up a bit.

- **Skinny belts** have the same effect as small sunglasses. Beware.

- **The quintessential bohemian outfit** of flowy dress + braided belt slung low on the hips looks good on almost everyone and is perfect for hot summer days.

- **A brightly colored belt** can spice up even the most basic outfit (red patent leather over a black blazer is a classic and sexy combination).

- **Almost anything can be used as a belt**—scarves, neckties, pretty strips of fabric, chain necklaces, spaghetti al dente—be creative!

Amazingly enough, the pieces covered in this chapter represent merely the tip of the accessories iceberg. Whenever you're shopping, whether it be at the upscale boutique, the thrift store, or your mom's closet, keep an eye out for those small but important touches like fabric flower corsages, unique eyeglass frames, and pretty patterned headbands. It's amazing what a tiny touch of colored silk or the glimmer of a silver necklace can do for an outfit—such little extras make the difference between looking good and looking unforgettable.

My advice? Be bold. Be unpredictable. Be a trendsetter. See the world through heart-shaped sunglasses. Make a pink fedora your trademark. Wear pearls to a chicken coop. Trust me, even the chickens will consider you a rare bird.

NINE

Work It:

HOW TO DRESS FOR THE JOB YOU WANT, THE JOB YOU HATE, AND EVERY JOB IN BETWEEN

ONCE UPON A TIME, I moved from Portland, Oregon, to Washington, DC, to work for a magazine. Up until then I worked as a freelance writer, and I had cultivated a personal style that was something like comfy bohemian meets chic fashion writer meets raccoon (I love shiny baubles). My only other foray into the world of traditional work wear had been during a yearlong stint as a receptionist. I had dressed like a bloated discount version of Carrie Bradshaw, but I had a supervisor so cool that when the sourpuss office manager asked, "Are you aware that your employee is wearing a tutu?" my boss replied, "Yes. And?"

Naturally, I assumed my free-spirited writer look would translate seamlessly to my new Real Job. Compounding my ignorance was the fact that the magazine had a science and nature focus, and having grown up around socially awkward scientists (my mom worked at the zoo and my dad at a primate research facility), I was confident that *anything* I wore would be better than stained jeans and button-up denim shirts—the unofficial uniform of scientists and zoologists worldwide.

STYLE LESSON #32:

Don't measure your work clothes against a zoologist's. No good can come of it.

When my first day of work rolled around, I sprang out of bed, eager to assemble the perfect introductory outfit. A blue silk dress and black tights sounded marvelous—how young, classic, and carefree!—but when I looked in the mirror, the whole thing seemed wrong. The dress was short, making it more girls'-night-out than business casual, and I hadn't taken into account the humidity of my new locale, so my legs were already sweating profusely beneath my black tights.

My second attempt included a black cardigan and a blue patterned bubble skirt. Again, when I looked in the mirror, it was all wrong. The bubble skirt was fun and hip, but too fun and hip for a first day, and the cardigan—a trusty standby in my freelance life—was, upon closer inspection, plagued with pilling and snags. I started to sweat for reasons other than the heat. Everywhere I looked there were cool, crazy clothes for a cool, crazy life—pink miniskirts in the closet, funky old man sweaters on the shelf, neon yellow jeans I'd purchased on a whim in the drawer—but few pieces worked together, and absolutely nothing seemed right for nine to five. And speaking of nine, the clock was ticking toward tardiness while I stood there in my shaping underwear, desperately trying to figure out if there was a way to make a gold sequined tunic business casual. Answer: No, there isn't.

STYLE LESSON #33:

There are a few pieces of clothing that can transition successfully from the nightclub to the office; a gold sequined tunic is not one of them.

I finally dug up a white cotton skirt (tucked away in my suitcase, no less) and paired it with a black V-neck tee and cute flats. Under normal circumstances I would have thrown on a big, shiny necklace (or three), but I was stricken with fashion paralysis and decided against it. I headed out the door, feeling basically presentable but devoid of style and personality. Just the way you want to feel on your first day, right?

When I arrived at the office, I met my new boss, one of the best-dressed women I'd ever encountered, all flouncy dress and high heels without a trace of zoologist. "Surely a fluke," I said to myself, but as I went around, meeting my new coworkers, it became obvious that button-up denim shirts were few and far between. While shaking hands with yet another sharply dressed editor, I looked down at my wrinkled skirt and scuffed flats and felt distinctly out of my league.

THE WORK CLOTHES CONUNDRUM

I love to express myself through my clothes. It's one of my favorite things about fashion, and getting dressed every morning is, for me, an introspective adventure. Am I feeling grumpy and mysterious? Then I'll reach for tough boots and a smear of black eyeliner. Did I wake up as bright and cheery as my hot pink raincoat? Then I'll throw it on, whether or not there's a severe drought. I think the personal nature of clothing is one of the unspoken reasons that dressing for work can be so difficult. Sure, there are the logistical issues like keeping cleavage in check and finding comfortable yet appropriate shoes, but figuring out how to dress in a professional way while remaining true to your own style is no small feat.

There's a big difference between having an awesome wardrobe and having awesome outfits to wear to work. You could have a cool new haircut (check), a vintage crocodile tote bag (check), and a closet overflowing with stylish clothes you adore (check), yet still find that dressing for a five-day workweek is not feasible.

After that first day, I shopped frantically to amass the basics of an appropriate work wardrobe. My bank account took a formidable hit, and my purchases were all over the map, from black blazers to printed skirts to zebra-patterned hoodies (oops), but I learned a few things in the process:

➤ **START WITH THE BASICS.** Use simple, complementary pieces as a foundation, and then add bolder, statement-making clothes. It's a good idea to invest in the pieces, such as black pants, that form the base of many outfits. Buy a couple pairs of quality trousers that fit well and age well, rather than twenty mediocre pairs that pill, tear, or make swishy sounds when you walk.

➤ **A LIGHTWEIGHT, EXTRA-LONG SWEATER** can be worn all year and looks good with literally everything. Throw on one of these, some pants if you're feeling ambitious, and you're ready for work.

➤ **YOU HAVE TO HAVE A GOOD BAG.** That stained leather satchel you found in your mom's closet is not whimsically bohemian, it's just plain old and not something you want to carry your lunch to work in (unfortunately I speak from experience).

➤ **SHOW YOUR PERSONALITY AND STYLE** with unique accessories. A knotted silk scarf, a double-wrap leather belt, an oversized brooch—accessories should be your new best friends.

The Bare-Bones Basics: Twelve Things Every Working Girl Simply Must Own

➤ **Black trousers** (good quality, right fit, classic style)

➤ **Knee-length skirt**

➤ **A few basic tank tops or T-shirts** (for layering)

➤ **Collared shirt or printed blouse**

➤ **Lightweight cardigan**

➤ **Slim-fitting V-neck,** scoop neck, or turtleneck sweater

➤ **Dark denim jeans**

➤ **Pretty raincoat** (can be worn over just about anything)

➤ **Classic wool coat** in a neutral color like white, black, or brown

➤ **Flat shoes**

➤ **Mid-height heels**

➤ **A medium to large handbag** in your preferred color

Second Tier: Indispensable Once You Own Them, but Not Absolutely Necessary

➤ **Black trousers one size too big** (for the day after the night you sample everything on the happy hour menu)

➤ **Pencil skirt**

➤ **Blouses with fun details** (like ruffles, a bow at the neck, or polka dots)

➤ **High heels**

➤ **Black or brown boots** (with or without a heel, depending on your personal preference)

➤ **Belt** (wear it OVER your button-up blazer or cardigan to be the cutest gal in the meeting)

➤ **Shirtdress** (with cardigan, tights, and mid-height pumps)

➤ **Vest** (button-up or V-neck pullover)

➤ **Neckties** (raid the men's sections at thrift stores to add a dose of androgyny to your office look)

➤ **Jewelry—lots and lots and lots of jewelry.** Try necklaces with large pendants, delicate gold or silver chains, dangly earrings, a string of pearls, brooches, bangles, charm bracelets, oversized rings, or pretty clips for your hair.

If you're on a budget and/or hastily assembling a work-appropriate wardrobe, do as I did and hit up affordable stores and sale racks. Play your cards right, and you can score a pair of pants, a skirt, a cardigan, and a coat for less than $150. But don't even attempt to thrift shop for your basics; it's too unreliable. Leave thrifting for the fun extras, like jewelry and gold sequined tunics.

THE THREE MOST COMMON WORK CLOTHES TRAPS AND HOW TO AVOID THEM

Like the Sirens awaiting Odysseus, there are three traps awaiting every woman as she gets dressed for work each morning. They are:

1. Revealing too much

2. Dressing too casually

3. Dressing uncomfortably

Let's break these down one at a time:

Revealing Too Much

What with the freedom modern day women have to wear whatever we want, plus the onslaught of super-high heels, skintight pants, effective push-up bras, and sheer fabrics, it's all too easy to get sucked into wearing club clothes to work. No matter how much you love your black mini-skirt and low-cut tank top, remember that throwing on a cardigan does not make the outfit work appropriate. As an added incentive, think how pleasantly surprised the hot IT guy will be when you show up at the holiday party in a strapless cocktail dress—if you've been wearing strapless cocktail dresses to work every day, the effect will be significantly dulled.

Be mindful of accidental exhibitionist tendencies as well. A friend of mine began her first day as a high school teacher wearing a brand-new outfit. She was feeling fabulous until she caught a good glimpse of herself in a window right before stepping into class. Apparently, her new pants were not only lightweight and flowy, but completely see-through. Worried about traumatizing her students with flashes of underwear, she spent the whole day sitting down behind her desk—not the best way to start the school year.

In addition, avoid long red fingernails and super-high heels for work, and review the law of trajectory (see diagram): that shirt you're wearing that seems perfectly modest? How about when your boss walks in while you're sitting down at a desk?

$$A^2 + B^2 = \text{SEE CLEAVAGE}$$

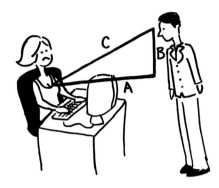

Dressing Too Casually

If you're worried that an outfit might be too casual for work, it is. Err on the side of put-together and professional. I'll discuss this approach in more detail later on, when I get into the whole "dress for the job you want" business, but one way to avoid inadvertently casual work days is to have a go-to work outfit at the ready. We're all human: sometimes we stay out until 3 a.m. on a weeknight, sometimes we fall asleep watching Japanese game shows and forget to do the laundry. Whatever the reason, there will come a time in your life (if not a few times a week, in your life) when you wake up late, panicked, and completely unprepared. Such mornings are when you're most at risk of throwing on whatever clothing you find on the floor, hoping your lady parts are covered, and booking it to the office. However, if you've tucked away some stretchy black pants and a flattering long sweater for just such an occasion, you'll look confident and cool and stand a good chance of being promoted above the guy who showed up, bleary-eyed, in jeans and a Little League T-shirt.

Dressing Uncomfortably

I once wore a pair of old tights to work, and all day they slipped and sagged and the waistband dug into my stomach and it just wasn't pretty. I spent most of the day sneaking off to the bathroom to conduct heroic hosiery adjustments, and then I went home.

You have to be comfortable to do good work, unless your job is testing uncomfortable clothes.

Buy clothes that fit, fabrics that have a bit of stretch, and shoes you can actually walk in. Repeat after me: women who claim that five-inch heels are comfortable are liars. A five-inch heel will give you a blister and a sprained ankle on your first trip to the copy machine.

Dressing uncomfortably doesn't only encompass the physical. Ideally, you should also feel emotionally comfortable in your work clothes, which means wearing things that make you feel confident, happy, and secure. Don't buy a bunch of structured blazers if they make you feel like a kid playing dress up. Don't wear pumps to the office if they make you feel insecure. If traditional suits just aren't your thing, find a softer alternative, like a pretty knee-length skirt with a short-sleeved blouse. Your work clothes should make you feel good about your appearance and yourself.

BUY ONE NEW PIECE EACH SEASON THAT MAKES YOU HAPPY TO GO TO WORK AND CONTINUE LIVING

No matter how awesome your job, the daily grind can get you down. So it's very important to reward yourself every now and again with a fashionable treat. Not only will this keep your morale up, but it will keep your professional wardrobe current. It's a total win-win. Except for your bank account, I guess, but hey, you're working hard! You deserve it! Just think about how much easier it will be to jump out of bed at 6:30 a.m. if you know a fresh pair of cool boots or soft new cashmere sweater awaits. Refer to The Splurge-a-Month Calendar for ideas and inspiration.

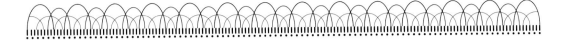

THE SPLURGE-A-MONTH CALENDAR

January
Handbag (try red!)

February
Showstopping necklace
and/or earrings

March
Spring coat in the season's
hottest color

April
Peep-toe pumps

May
Swingy skirt in a bold
color or fun pattern

June
Oversized (and overpriced)
sunglasses

July
Sexy bra and panties to
wear under your work
clothes

August
Silk blouse

September
A great-fitting blazer

October
Boots

November
Cashmere sweater

December
A new rainbow array of
tights

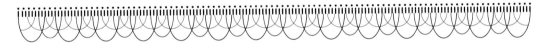

BUT WHAT ABOUT SUITS?

Suits are tricky. When done well, they are flattering, simple, and can elevate your look along with your job prospects; when done wrong, they can lead people to ask you for a shrimp cocktail. It's important to consider the cut and color, as well as the fit, of a prospective suit. There's nothing worse than a baggy suit except a too-tight suit. Try on at least a few options until you find one that works for you.

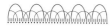

Navy blue suit with three-quarter-length skirt says, "Right this way to your table, folks."

Hot pink suit jacket with bustier and miniskirt says, "I'm a working girl . . . in the oldest profession in the world!"

Pastel pantsuit says, "Can I count on your vote?"

Blue suit with fitted, flared blazer and flared skirt says, "In the event of a water landing, your seat cushion may also be used as a flotation device."

Nice-fitting black suit says, "I had to turn down three promotions just last week!"

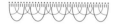

Alternatives to the Suit

Let's talk about the faux suit. The faux suit looks like a suit, talks like a suit, and may even have a fake ID listing its name as Suit, but it's not a suit; it's two separates, which means you probably already have the makings in your closet.

A few faux suit examples:

➤ **A pair of black pants** you love paired with a fitted blazer and chunky belt.

➤ **A white skirt** with a retro black swing jacket.

➤ **A pair of pinstriped pants,** crisp white shirt, and solid blazer.

➤ **A pencil skirt** with a cropped tweed jacket.

Using items already in your wardrobe lets you step up your professional look without spending a ton of money. The possibilities are endless, and if you do make a new purchase or two, the faux suit allows you to buy tops and bottoms in different sizes for a better fit.

WHAT TO WEAR IF . . .

You're Trying to Get a Promotion

You know the old adage "Dress for the job you want"? Well, it's sort of true. Dress like a homeless person, and you'll probably score a pink slip. Wear a clown suit every day, and chances are you'll be recruited by a traveling circus. So if you're looking to rise professionally, dress in a manner that allows the higher-ups to envision you in that role.

Say you've been working an entry-level position at a large company. You dress barely as nicely as required—maybe your daily uniform is a collared shirt and dark jeans—so your coworkers and bosses see you as an entry-level worker. What would they see if you started dressing in wool trousers and blazers instead?

About ten years ago, a friend of mine supervised a group of employees who were just out of college and getting their professional starts. The vast majority of the group dressed like they were just out of college, or maybe still in it: T-shirts, wrinkled pants, Birkenstocks, and messy hair seemed to be the daily uniform of choice, which was fine, since the office environment was decidedly informal. But there was one young woman in the group who came to work every day in a fitted suit and heels and with her hair in a pretty bun. She wasn't necessarily more talented or qualified than her coworkers, but she dressed like she was and ended up being promoted so quickly that her wrinkled pants–wearing peers barely got a chance to know her. Today, that young woman is probably your boss.

Now, how does this advice apply if you're one of the many people who work for a cool Internet company, where the dress code is "Wear pants, most days" and the CEO dons a T-shirt and flip-flops to play putt-putt golf in the lobby? Well, dressing professionally isn't just about the way others see you, it's about how you see yourself. I know I feel more put-together when I look more put-together, and that state of mind makes me more productive at work. Wearing your pajamas to the office is fun for a while, but do me a favor and try a pencil skirt tomorrow. Dress for the job you deserve.

You're Trying to Get Laid Off So You Can Travel

Try concert T-shirts, socks with sandals, and hold off on the showers and personal hygiene. With any luck, when it's time to downsize, you'll be the first on the boss's list.

You're the Receptionist

Being a receptionist is such a great excuse to wear fun '60s-style clothes—pencil skirts, box jackets with oversized buttons, pretty hosiery, and peep-toe pumps. Sure, it's cliché, but when cliché involves cat eye glasses, I'm totally fine with it.

You're the Boss

Always dress a little nicer than you think you have to: rock the fitted suits, collared shirts, wide leg pants, high heels, and authoritative equestrian boots.

You're the Creative Art Director

Fashion magazines almost always have editorial spreads dedicated to work clothes, and these spreads make most women exclaim, "Who in the hell can actually go to work in an oversized designer blazer and vintage wedding dress?" Well, no one can, but if you're the creative art director, you probably come closest. Women in creative fields often have much more flexibility with their style choices than their business casual peers, and taking fashion risks can be a way to literally wear your creativity on your sleeve. Go for bold colors and statement-making jewelry. Scope out boutiques for unique shoes with brag-worthy backstories ("Oh these old things? They were made by a shoe shaman in the Middle East, who only makes three shoes a year. I suppose I was lucky to score the complete pair.").

You're Required to Wear Scrubs to Work and You Have to Wear Sneakers Because You're on Your Feet All Day and Is There Any Hope of Being Stylish?

Not really, but that's OK. Get a great haircut to direct the focus to your face, steer clear of scrubs emblazoned with miniature animals or holiday themes, and commit to bringing your fashion A-game to evenings and weekends.

You're Headed from Work to Happy Hour

It is shockingly easy to transition from a simple work ensemble to a cute outfit for socializing. Throw some shiny jewelry, high heels, and a pretty camisole into your work bag in the morning. At the end of your workday, swap out your practical shoes for the high heels, put the camisole on under your jacket, add the shiny jewelry to whatever ornaments you're already wearing (there's no such thing as too much!), and ta-da, you're ready! One more piece of advice: beware of Casual Friday. Friday is the day you're most likely to receive an invitation to head straight from work to a social engagement, and there's nothing worse than showing up to a hot new restaurant in yoga pants and a fleece covered in cat hair.

WORK IT OUT

Sure, it can be annoying, but the office dress code makes us put a little more thought into how we present ourselves to the world, and that is never a bad thing. If we didn't have to go to work, we might not push ourselves to create styles that are both professional and all our own; we might all wear our college sweatshirts and ripped jeans every day. All skills improve with practice, and I can't think of a better fashion training exercise than putting together attractive, comfortable, and presentable outfits five (way too early) mornings a week. The style savvy you gather and build in your work life will undoubtedly improve the way you dress in your off-the-clock life.

Every decade of working women has had a signature style, from the shift dresses of the '60s to the power suits of the '80s. What will our generation be wearing when we change the world? On Monday morning, you get to decide.

 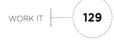

TEN

Around the World in 80 Outfits:

HOW TO CRAM YOUR STYLE INTO A SUITCASE, A WORKOUT BAG, OR AN ITTY-BITTY BIKINI

I HAIL FROM OREGON, where people dress in high-performance outdoor gear for dinner at a classy restaurant, because apparently you never know when you might need to head out on an eighty-mile cycling trip. I think my upbringing sparked my initial interest in fashion, actually; I was the little girl looking out at the fir trees beyond her bedroom window, daydreaming about faraway lands where people wore high heels.

While I was raised in an area where function always conquered fashion, many people grew up in places where fashion always won. Hopefully this chapter, covering workout gear, travel clothing, and (gasp!) swimsuits, will help you dress for those occasions when function and fashion must shake hands and agree to get along.

FIRST UP, WORKOUT WEAR

I've been a dedicated workout contrarian since middle school. My seventh grade gym teacher was a documented sadist (well, I once wrote, "Mr. Alley is a sadist" in my notebook), who would force us out to the track for long runs in the summer heat, set up a lawn chair and a glass of lemonade for himself, and say things like, "Sorry, I can't record your mile time because I only have a stopwatch, not a sundial." Looking back, maybe he was kind of clever, but still, I spent many hours of my adolescence organizing an anti-hustle movement (the hugely successful Twenty-Minute Mile Club) and searching for legal precedents to sue over forced physical activity (never did find anything).

Unfortunately, this attitude has stuck with me into adulthood, leaving me unable to enjoy the services of a personal trainer ("Hustle!" she would say, and I would say, "NO!"), or even look at a jogger without becoming hostile—"OK! I get it! You're better than me! You can run more than fifty feet without needing a lung transplant and only the right parts of you are bouncing and I'M SO SLOW!" Yes, I should probably go to therapy to work through my issues, but I've found that cute gym clothes are almost as effective. Nothing makes me want to go to the gym and get my hustle on more than some colorful sneakers, high-tech workout pants, or a bright yellow headband.

STYLE LESSON #35:

You don't have to buy a whole new wardrobe just for working out, but don't make it obvious that you didn't.

I know, I know, this sounds like a particularly convoluted Yogi Berra quote, but here's what I mean: you absolutely do not have to spend thousands of dollars on new, brand-name, super-cool workout gear, but if you go to the gym every day in a baggy "2001 Smith Family Reunion: *Gettin' Smithy Wit' It!*" T-shirt, people will quickly get wise to your dirty, repetitive ways. There's not anything explicitly wrong with wearing old T-shirts to work out (I'm guilty of it on occasion), but there's nothing right about it either. I believe that it's always a good idea to put a little effort into your look, whether you're going to the gym or high tea with the queen. When you exercise, you're doing something great for your body, so why not make a commitment to looking good *while* you do it? An added incentive: it seems to be a law of physics that you only run into people you know when you look your worst. When I used to wear too-short spandex shorts and bawdy message T-shirts to the gym (it was a phase), there was a 100 percent chance that I'd see one of my coworkers or ex-boyfriends. If that's not a motivating excuse to put a little effort into your workout clothes, I don't know what is.

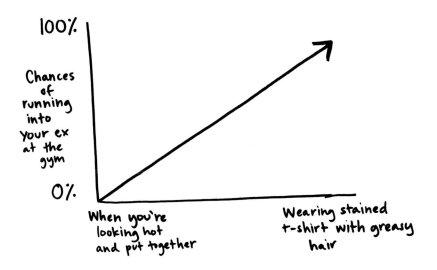

Some General Tips on Dressing for the Gym

➤ **YOGA IS PERHAPS** the most stylish form of exercise ever invented. Any piece of clothing meant for yoga is usually cute enough to go from yoga to cardio to grocery store.

➤ **I'M A HUGE FAN OF '70S-INSPIRED WORKOUT GEAR**—nylon running shorts in fun colors, cotton kneesocks, and mesh tank tops. Try not to wear more than one of these items at the same time, though, or you'll end up looking like a hipster party guest.

*No. Unless your everyday
style is sporty enough to
carry off a nylon Nike
bag, just use the gym as
an excuse to get another
awesome oversized bag.
I like big tote bags in
bright colors. Get one
large enough and nice
enough to carry to work
on those days you want
to head straight from the
office to the gym. The
world doesn't need to
know you're carrying
smelly shoes.*

➤ **STRETCHY BLACK PANTS ARE FLATTERING ON EVERYONE.** If you have yet to find a pair that looks good on you, go to a store with a large athletic department or one that specializes in women's workout apparel, and try on every style—cropped, flared, tapered, straight, detailed, and plain. I assure you, you'll walk (or jog) out of there with some awesome, flattering new pants.

➤ **WEAR COLOR ON THE PART OF YOUR BODY** you want to accentuate. If you're bottom heavy, rock those black pants and add a colorful tank top. If you like your legs more, try pink shorts with a black shirt.

➤ **IF YOU HAVE LONG HAIR,** wear it up in a ponytail or bun. Long, sweaty hair sticking to your face = uncomfortable and unattractive.

➤ **WHILE YOU SHOULD PUT SOME EFFORT INTO YOUR EXERCISE LOOK,** be wary of crossing over into trying-too-hard territory—loads of makeup, super-low-cut tops, and short shorts aren't exactly conducive to a good workout.

Which everyday clothes work for the gym, which gym clothes work for everyday, and which work for both?

GYM
- sports bras
- running shoes
- white socks
- spandex shorts
- spandex anything
- sweatbands and wristbands
- sweatbands
- anything sweaty

BOTH
- plain tank tops
- stretchy black pants
- nylon jacket
- 70s running shorts
- anything yoga

EVERYDAY
- dresses
- lace bras and panties
- jeans
- anything polyester or acrylic
- lipstick
- nylons and hosiery
- fake nails

A Word About Sports Bras

I have a friend who, when she played high school basketball in the late '80s, had no idea there was such a thing as a sports bra. A few years after graduating, she was home over the holidays when an old buddy revealed that everyone at school had called her "Bouncy" behind her back. Ever since, my friend's been something of a sports bra connoisseur/vigilante. She owns ten of them and delivers impassioned lectures to her well-endowed friends on the grave importance of the sports bra. As someone who has also been called "Bouncy" (even when wearing a sports bra), I'm in complete agreement.

STYLE LESSON #36:

If you are a B cup or larger, invest in a couple of good sports bras. It could save you from a lifelong nickname of "Bouncy."

Try a variety of styles and jump around in the dressing room to make sure they're secure. Look for ones with cups, underwires, or at least two clearly separated compartments—the single boob loaf look is almost worse than the bouncy look. I said almost.

OUTDOOR RECREATION: THE CALL OF THE WILD

I've been hiking since I was a kid. My family favored fast-paced death marches up steep terrain, with my mom in the lead shouting, "Stragglers will be left behind!" my dad and two dutiful brothers keeping pace, and my youngest, more dramatic brother and me about half a mile back, shuffling along and moaning, "We are actually going to DIE." I wish I could say I have matured measurably since then, but that would be a lie.

What to Wear on the Trail

When putting together your hiking outfit, utilize those items that overlap everyday life and gym clothes. Ribbed tank tops, stretchy black pants, and fleece pullovers all work great for hiking, and most people have them in their wardrobes already.

Here are some other pieces that will serve you well on the trail:

➤ **Hoodie**

➤ **Long-sleeved crewneck tee**

➤ **Heavy, warm fleece**

➤ **Cool, flattering rain jacket** (does exist)

➤ **Cool, flattering rain pants** (a little harder to find)

➤ **Black jersey skirt** (wear spandex shorts underneath)

➤ **Kneesocks** (double bonus: repel ticks and make legs look slim!)

➤ **Cargo pants** (Hiking may be one of the only times in your life when you can wear these without making people wonder if you are a time traveler from the mid-'90s.)

When pondering your hiking outfit, be sure to answer this important philosophical question: *What are you doing after the hike*? Feel free to throw on a grungy T-shirt if the plan is just to be at one with nature, but make sure your friends aren't wanting to do a post-hike celebration at the bar, or your mom isn't planning to get professional family photos taken (my mom actually did this once—everyone who received our Christmas card commented, "The kids are so grown up! And sweaty!").

Layering

When you're exercising out in the wild, you have to shield yourself from the sun, the cold, the rain, and blood-sucking insects (what's the upside of hiking again?), so it makes sense to begin your hike tightly swathed in high-tech protective fabrics. Twenty minutes into the hike, however, you may find yourself sweating profusely, tearing off your sensible long-sleeved shirt, and screaming, "Bring it on, mosquitoes!" This is why mastering the art of outdoor layering is so important.

Hiking is sort of like strip poker: by the end, all the participants are hot, sweaty, and nearly naked, and the winner is the person who wore the most layers.

The key to layering is making sure all of your layers are light and thin. You want each article of clothing to serve its purpose (keep you warm, keep you dry, stop bullets, etc.) without weighing you down. There's nothing worse than having to abandon a $300 down jacket on the side of the trail, no matter how much a stylish bear might appreciate it.

Master a basic layering scheme, and you'll be able to put together effective outfits for not just hiking, but camping, beach trips, weekends in the mountains, and other outdoorsy activities as well. Teach your friends a few layering techniques too, and your next strip poker game could last for days.

TRAVELING

Here's the thing about traveling: it's always good. Even the "bad" parts of traveling—like getting off at the wrong subway stop or losing a foot to piranhas—are good, because they add to our life experiences and give us impressive stories to tell strangers at bars. Dressing badly while you explore the world won't necessarily make your trip less enjoyable (well, an epic blister might), but dressing well can only enhance the experience.

What to Wear in the Air

Fashion magazines love to talk about the perfect plane outfit, which, according to them, consists of expensive jeans, a long-sleeved shirt, and a bright pashmina wrap (they really go crazy over the pashmina—"use it as a scarf at the airport and a blanket on the plane! AMAZING!").

I used to heed this advice; I tried to be cute on plane rides, I really did. I loved the idea of landing in a new place all fresh and chic and ready to roll. But in reality, my intense fear of flying means that my hours in the air are spent hyperventilating, brainstorming creative ways to end my life with a complimentary beverage cup, and screaming, "Gah! This is it! We're going down! Good-bye cruel world!" once every five minutes or so. By the time I arrive at my destination, I've gone hoarse, lost all the color in my face, contracted a cold, and I just want to sleep for days on the sweet, sweet ground.

These are the times in my life when I probably care the least about being cute.

In addition, I've never found jeans to be particularly comfortable on plane rides. I've worn expensive jeans, cheap jeans, tight jeans, and loose jeans, and they always end up sticking to me or bunching up wrong or being too stiff or cutting into my stomach, and it's enough to make me very nearly condone velour tracksuits. But not quite.

STYLE LESSON #38:

When choosing your outfit for a plane ride, choose comfort over style, but please don't choose a pink velour tracksuit.

I'm only hating on the tracksuit because it's so predictable—take a trip to the Vegas airport and you'll think you've stumbled upon a velour tradeshow. I do, however, suggest wearing whatever feels comfortable and right for you, whether that means some hip-hop-style sweats slung low on your hips with a tank top and hoodie, or jeans and a cashmere sweater, or maybe a pashmina wrapped around your nude body. I usually go with black leggings and a long sweater. It might make me look like an '80s backup dancer, but it's the most I can muster when I'm convinced I am going to die.

What to Wear on (Foreign) Land

If comfort is the most important factor when considering your in-flight outfit, "simplicity" should be your mantra when packing your suitcase. Most people understand the stereotypical tourist fashion sins and leave their fanny packs at home, but trying too hard can make you look just as foolish. If you've never worn high heels, walking around Paris in them for eight hours is probably not the best way to learn.

I'm one of those people who, when packing for a trip, digs around in the back of my closet for my coolest, wildest clothes that I never wear in my normal life, convinced "Traveling Winona" is cool enough to wear them. Upon arriving at my destination, I am horrified to realize "Traveling Winona" doesn't actually exist, and I'm stuck with a suitcase full of tie-dyed maxi dresses and sheer club shirts.

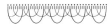

FIVE THINGS THAT SCREAM "TOURIST"

Screaming, "I'm a tourist!"

Fanny packs, backpacks

White sneakers

Large, messily folded maps

Spraining your ankle in super-high heels while trying to impress the Euro-girls

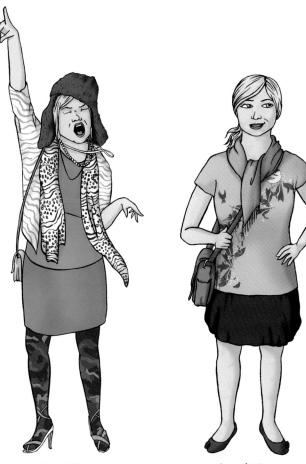

Traveling Winona 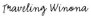   *Actual Winona*

If you don't wear your leopard-print trench coat here, you will not wear it in Europe.

When you travel, bring along your favorite, simplest outfits: the great-fitting dark denim jeans and cream cardigan, the flowy yellow skirt and brown tank top, the perfect jersey sundress. Choose coordinating pieces you wear often and feel good in.

To mix things up without taking up precious suitcase space, bring a standout accessory and make it your traveling trademark. Better yet, bring one and buy a couple more during your trip. Here are some ideas:

➤ **Colorful scarf**

➤ **Slouchy hat**

➤ **Oversized sunglasses**

➤ **Red lipstick**

➤ **Pretty ribbon sash**

➤ **Striped tote bag**

Globe-trotting without Getting Blisters

Which shoes you throw in your suitcase is the most important decision of your entire trip, with the possible exception of whether or not to accept a local's generous offer of fried goat brains (Hello, good bar story!). Traveling usually involves massive amounts of walking, so a little pinch or a minor blister can quickly blossom into a severe problem. As my wise friend Molly once said, "Slowly filling up your shoe with blood is no way to travel."

You don't want to become a sad stereotype and wear gym shoes to pose in front of the Eiffel Tower, but you also don't want to go home with scarred stumps where your feet used to be. It can be tough to find shoes that meet the stringent criteria, but low wedges, cushioned ballet flats, thick-soled sandals, and trusty worn-in boots are great options. Check out the following lists for more info.

LOOK FOR:

➤ **Cushioning . . . lots and lots of cushioning:** I tend to think my basic flats will be just fine for a day of walking, but after an hour, I'm feeling every tiny pebble beneath my feet. Look for shoes that have a lot of inner cushioning.

➤ **A thick sole:** Because nothing ruins a trip faster than a rusty nail through your foot.

➤ **A low heel:** Unless you wear high heels every day and genuinely feel more comfortable in them than in flats, it's best to stick with a small (lower than one inch) heel.

➤ **Simplicity:** Again with the simplicity, I know, but the fewer straps, zippers, and buckles a shoe has, the lesser the chances of straps snapping, zipper rubbing, or buckles breaking.

➤ **Overall quality:** Quality shoes might cost a little more, but they last longer and are kinder to your feet.

AVOID:

➤ **Open toes:** If you want to keep your toes, that is.

➤ **Stilettos:** Wear these in Europe, and watch the locals laugh as you teeter around cobblestoned streets; wear them in South America, and watch the locals laugh as you sink into the dirt. (Unless you are in Buenos Aires, of course. In that case, tango!)

➤ **Brand-new shoes:** Even if they're labeled "SUPER COMFORT PLUS," and even if you've owned the exact same style before, the first few wearings can be awkward and painful. Definitely buy new shoes for your trip, but break them in before you leave.

SWIMSUITS: TIME TO DITCH THE BLACK SUIT

I do not have, and have never had, what you would call a flat stomach. I've owned one bikini in my life, when I was five years old, and in it I bore a striking resemblance to a young, blond John Goodman. For most of my adult life, my summers have included conservative black one-piece swimsuits that didn't match my personality at all. I was trying to camouflage my stomach, but I looked like I was going to a pool funeral.

One summer, a few years ago, I tinkered with the idea of finally conquering my mortal fear of bikinis and just going for it. I felt it would be a great showing of body confidence, like, "Yes, I have a big belly, but I'm in a bikini and I'm proud!" Plus, as every woman knows, bikinis are *always* cuter than one-pieces. I've seen that trend change for the better recently (like in the "A Swimsuit for EVERY Body" sections of the summer fashion magazines, where they actually now have pages devoted to hot one-piece suits instead of the usual, "Bikini not for you? Just kill yourself."), but it's still pretty slim pickings out there.

I found a cute bikini online (it didn't take long), but as my cursor hovered over the "Add to Cart" button, I froze. My cool, brave, body-confident bikini plan had some kinks in it. Mainly, I was way too scared to buy a bikini.

I decided my time would be better spent attempting to find a truly unique, truly flattering, truly not black-and-boring one-piece suit. I needed something that celebrated my body type and made me feel good about myself. Could it be done? At first, it sure didn't seem like it. I scoured magazines, stores, and Web sites; pretty much all the suits recommended for rounder women were not only black and boring, but came with names like "Instant Slenderizer" or "Fat-Belly-B-Gone" or "Waterproof Corset." Not exactly positive, self-loving stuff.

I was about to give up and become one of those sad people who swims in a baggy T-shirt, pretending it's by choice ("I just *love* baggy T-shirts!") rather than for lack of flattering swimsuit options, but then I found it. It was on a little Web site in the corner of the Internet—a retro sheath swimsuit with low-cut legs, ruching at the waist, and a sweetheart neckline and halter straps. Almost identical to what Marilyn Monroe wore in many a beach photo shoot, it was absolutely perfect—stylish, attention grabbing, and totally flattering. I bought one in black-and-white polka dot, and another in red soon after. Now I like to lounge by the pool in my new suit and big black sunglasses and pretend I'm reading, but really I'm just pondering how anyone could possibly look more glamorous than I.

Seriously, there's a swimsuit for everyone.
Don't resort to the baggy T-shirt just yet.

How to Find the Suit for You

Everyone has read a swimsuit guide (or a hundred) that tells you how to hide your "worst" feature. I'm so sick of that attitude; it's what put me in pool funeral outfits for a large portion of my life. Here are some swimsuit suggestions to play up your best features:

If you love your . . .

LEGS

Try a suit with high-cut leg holes to show them off (even if you don't love your legs, high-cut leg holes are visually lengthening, so give them a try).

BELLY

Obviously, rock the bikini, but also think about a one-piece with cutout sides (if I put one of these on, it would look like my love handles were making a desperate bid for freedom) or a sporty tankini.

ARMS/SHOULDERS

A halter top is like a beautiful frame for your arms and upper body, and strapless suits are always a fun, tan line–free choice.

SKIN

If you have darker skin, try a light colored suit for a striking contrast (just make sure those white suits have linings . . .). Pale ladies look fantastic in dark colors and jewel tones (emerald green, deep blue, and dark purple).

General Tips for Shopping for Swimsuits

➤ **THE INTERNET WAS INVENTED** so you could order a mass of swimsuits, have them delivered to your house, and try them on one by one, with breaks to eat cake or drink heavily.

➤ **DON'T EVER RULE OUT A PARTICULAR STYLE OF SWIMSUIT.** There is a chance that someday I will find a bikini I like, and I will buy it, and I will wear it. The same goes for my friends who swear they will never wear a swim skirt. The same goes for you.

➤ **KEEP IN MIND WHAT YOU'RE ACTUALLY GOING TO BE DOING** in the swimsuit—there's a substantial difference between glamorous lounging and, like, competitive swimming. I once bought a suit that only looked good when I was lying down, and then I signed up for a junior lifeguarding class. Many of my practice victims drowned as I was trying to save them horizontally.

Sometimes, in life, you need to go swimming. Sometimes you need to drag your butt to the gym. Sometimes you need to max out your credit card and hop on a plane to Ibiza. What you wear for these activities and adventures isn't the most important thing, but looking great can certainly make you feel better as you move through life. You'll still burn calories at the gym if you're wearing a baggy family reunion T-shirt, but wouldn't you feel better in some cute workout gear? And yeah, hanging out by the pool in a somber black one-piece is fine, but a polka-dot turquoise tankini is much more fun! You could throw a silk baby doll dress in your suitcase when bound for Paris, or you could keep it simple and spend your time touring the Louvre instead of ironing in your hotel room. The choice is yours, but I think it's an easy one.

ELEVEN

How to Wear Your Fancy Pants:

DRESSING FOR DATES, WEDDINGS, AND OTHER SPECIAL OCCASIONS

WHEN I WAS ABOUT SEVEN, I MADE MY TELEVISION DEBUT. My dad took my brother and me to *The Ramblin' Rod Show*, a kids' TV program filmed in a neighboring town with a live studio audience. This is my first memory of a special occasion, an occasion that called for a special outfit.

The set consisted of a small arrangement of bleachers stocked with local children, who would cheer wildly when Rod introduced a new cartoon. Rod was a jovial, middle-aged man who wore a long brown vest covered in buttons and left ample time between each short cartoon to banter with the lucky kids sitting in the top row. The highlight of each show, however, was the Smile Contest, when the camera would pan over rows of kids grimacing with the determination and desperation that comes with knowing a sticker prize pack is on the line.

I knew I was going to win the Smile Contest, because I had a secret I'd been practicing in the mirror: if I pushed my tongue up against of the back of my top teeth ever so slightly, it shaped my mouth into an undeniably adorable grin. Plus, I didn't have braces.

My outfit though, that was to be the clincher—I chose a soft blue dress with a flared skirt and little red rosettes along the neckline. It looked so great with my white cable-knit tights and jelly sandals that I imagined as soon as I set foot in the studio, they'd call off the contest and declare me the winner. The night before the taping, I cleared a space on my bedroom wall where my new stickers would go.

When we got to the studio, my plan crumbled. The room was cold and sparse, and the producer had the audacity to seat me in the very bottom row next to my obnoxious brother. The good news was, my full outfit would be visible to the world; the bad news was, I was so nervous I could barely remember my name.

After an eternity of cartoons, Ramblin' Rod finally announced the start of the Smile Contest. Frantic, circus-style music started and the camera began its journey through the bleachers. "All right kids, let's see those smiles," he crooned. "Keep smilin'! Biiiiiiig grins, now!" As the lens settled on me, I was so tense with concentration on my tongue placement that I looked to have a severe case of lockjaw. On the tape, the camera operator lingers on my frozen face for a moment, perhaps wondering if I've had a stroke, as I stare intently at the concrete studio floor. Eventually, the camera moves along and my creepy visage is forgotten.

My brother won the Smile Contest. He was wearing paint-spattered MC Hammer pants and a racecar T-shirt.

Despite this emotional childhood trauma, dressing up for special occasions is one of my favorite activities. It's so much fun to put extra effort into your appearance and see how those around you react. Even though I went home without those sweet, sweet stickers, this Ramblin' Rod parable contains an important lesson concerning smile contests and special occasions in general: don't overthink it. Just be yourself.

DRESSING FOR A DATE

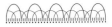

Let's start things off with one of the most exciting special occasions of all: the date. A friend of mine once said, "The best part of a date is getting ready for it." Wiser words were never spoken. We all know there are a million ways a date can go badly (stepping in dog waste, being set up with a guy who wears a monocle), but in the hours leading up to it, everything is perfect. Bask in the untainted anticipation while you primp and pamper yourself, and really have fun with the process of getting ready. This goes for women in long-term relationships as well—never give up on your pre-date ritual, even if you've been dating your date for thirty years. With that maxim in mind, here are my top three tips for dressing for first dates, last dates, and every date in between.

1. Be comfortable.

First and foremost, you have to feel good in the clothes you're wearing. Believe it or not, you don't look your best while pulling down the hem of your dress every five minutes or trying to subtly nurse a monster blister between cocktails. In the work chapter, I mentioned that you have to be comfortable to do good work; you also have to be comfortable to be a good date.

2. Be yourself.

This is especially important for first dates. If you normally wear ripped jeans and plain T-shirts, don't squeeze yourself into a bouncy pink dress for a date. A nice pair of jeans and a pretty blouse will look just as gorgeous and most importantly, you'll look and feel like you.

STYLE LESSON #41:

To avoid being sued for misrepresentation, don't dress up for a date as anyone but yourself.

THE SPECIAL OCCASIONS FORMALITY SPECTRUM

Ranked in order of least to greatest in formality and importance:

1.
First date

2.
Gallery opening/ night at the theater

3.
Birthday celebration at national chain Italian restaurant

4.
Office party

5.
Wedding (guest)

6.
Charity auction/ fundraiser

7.
Wedding (bridesmaid)

8.
Dinner with foreign heads of state

9.
Wedding (bride)

10.
Appearance on The Ramblin' Rod Show.

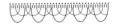

Haven't you seen all those romantic comedies where the main character claims to be a doctor or something, but they're actually not and then things get very complicated? Don't pretend to be a doctor.

My artist friend passed along some great advice given to her by one of her professors: "When you're meeting with a client, wear your dirty clothes, but take a shower." I think the dating version of this advice goes like so: when you're meeting with a potential lover, wear nicer versions of your normal clothes, and take a shower.

3. Don't be afraid of color.

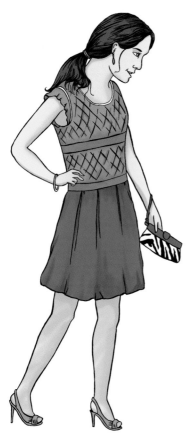

If black is truly your trademark, then rock the all-black outfit, but don't let it become your safe choice. Black may be slimming, but blue and red and green and purple are beautiful and memorable. Make a decision to stand out and see how it affects your mood and your date.

DRESSING FOR EVENTS

From *The Ramblin' Rod Show* to gallery openings to charity galas to parole hearings, a lady's life is full of special events that call for special outfits. The three guidelines I discussed in the dating section will serve you well at any special occasion, but here are three more tips for putting your best outfit forward:

1. Let your personal style, not the theme of the event, dictate your outfit.

I knew a girl in high school who had a shocking array of themed outfits, and would wear a sassy little Mrs. Claus suit to a holiday pancake breakfast, a sassy little cat dress to an animal shelter fundraiser, etc. While she surely had good intentions, her costumes made her look like the event's mascot rather than an enthusiastic attendee. Your formal clothes should be congruent with your everyday style. For dates *and* events, remember to dress like yourself, only better.

2. Don't wait to buy a formal dress until you need a formal dress.

Buy a formal dress when you find a formal dress you love. Trust me on this—shopping for formalwear at the last minute is the shopping stress equivalent of perusing the store while being stalked by a hungry tiger. You won't have any fun, you might not be happy with your hurried choice, and you'll probably spend too much money.

STYLE LESSON #42:

Make a habit of glancing at the formalwear sale racks when shopping for mundane things like jeans or unsalted butter, and you're sure to find an affordable gem that will have you itching for a formal invite to somewhere, anywhere!

3. Have a go-to special occasion outfit.

Growing up, one of my friend's moms kept a closet full of cute, generic, prewrapped gifts on the ready in case of forgotten birthdays or housewarming parties. I have yet to stumble upon another idea so brilliant, and I think the concept can easily be applied to formalwear. You should have a cute, generic, prewrapped outfit in your closet that you can throw on in the event of a last-minute, um, event.

Your go-to outfit doesn't need to be new or particularly flashy; it could be that cliché-but-fabulous Little Black Dress or a sleek pantsuit, but it must be easy and versatile. Don't forget the power of accessories here—throw on a simple, stylish base (like that LBD) for anything from a garden wedding to a presidential inauguration, and add opera gloves or flip-flops accordingly.

DRESSING ROOM DIARIES:
THE TROUBLE WITH VINTAGE

There is only one thing better than finding the perfect vintage dress to wear to an event, and that is getting a compliment on your perfect vintage dress and being able to say, "Oh, this? It's vintage."

The problem is, it's exceedingly difficult to find the perfect vintage dress. A dress has to fit correctly in about five different places, and the chances of this occurring in a garment that's five decades old are not so good. I have a few friends who wear nothing but vintage dresses and look absolutely stunning; I also have a lot of friends who try to wear vintage dresses and end up looking like they're borrowing clothes from an American Girl doll (I'm included in this group). Here's the deal: Do not wear a dress simply because it's cute and it's vintage; wear a dress because it fits you.

A few ways to avoid the American Girl doll vintage dress trap:

➤ **Never, ever buy a vintage dress** without trying it on. Sizes were so different back then, there might as well not be a number on the tag (and sometimes, there isn't).

➤ **Be honest with yourself**—does the dress actually look good on *you*, or are you blinded by its vintage charms?

➤ **Be a personal vintage dress shopper** for your friends. Often, when I stumble upon an amazing vintage find, I buy it impulsively out of love and then wear it because I bought it, even if it's a 1960s size 2. A much healthier alternative is to continue to buy these beautiful dresses impulsively out of love, but gift them to my teeny-tiny vintage-loving friends. This habit makes me popular and forces me to wait for a real vintage gem that's right for me.

➤ **If you're head over heels** for a dress that doesn't quite work on you, spend some money to get it altered. Take the waist in or out, have it hemmed, enlarge wrist openings, etc. Think about creative alterations too, like shortening a dowdy long dress into a mini, replacing buttons, or removing sleeves.

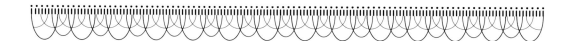

DRESSING FOR A WEDDING

Weddings are joyous occasions that tend to elicit stress and pain from everyone involved, but it doesn't have to be that way. A wedding is an opportunity to wear an amazing little dress and get your picture taken and flirt and dance and drink. Someone else is paying for the party, so have fun!

A Note to the Guest

Do me a favor, and don't complain about having to get dressed up to go to a wedding or not knowing what to wear to a wedding. Today's weddings are festive celebrations of love with free cake. Back in our grandmothers' and even our mothers' days, weddings were hard-core etiquette orgies where one minor faux pas could get you blacklisted for life (see list below for examples).

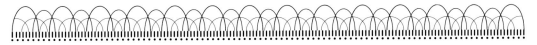

TEN WEDDING STYLE RULES FROM 1958
(WITH UPDATED COMMENTARY)

1. ~~DON'T~~ WEAR BLACK. *But to keep from appearing drab, look for fun details like embroidery, a voluminous skirt, or a ribbon sash.*

2. DON'T WEAR WHITE. *I guess I kind of agree with this one, but only because white is sort of boring. Wear pink or green or yellow or blue instead.*

3. WEAR A ~~HAT~~ FEATHERED HEADBAND! *These are soooo pretty, and they won't block anyone's view.*

4. DON'T OUTSHINE THE BRIDE. *As long as you don't consciously try to look prettier than her, or wear a dress that gives a clear view of your privates, you're probably OK.*

5. PICK BRIDESMAIDS ~~YOUNGER THAN YOU WHO ARE NOT MARRIED.~~ *however the hell you want to— I fully intend to have my three brothers standing next to me on my wedding day.*

6. ALWAYS WEAR NYLONS AND CLOSED-TOED PUMPS *if you are dressing up as an old lady for Halloween.*

7. ~~NEVER~~ WEAR FLOWERS IN YOUR HAIR ~~IF YOU ARE NOT IN THE WEDDING PARTY.~~ *any chance you get!*

8. CALL THE BRIDE AHEAD OF TIME AND ASK ~~WHAT THE COLOR THEME IS SO YOU CAN MATCH YOUR DRESS.~~ *when would be a good time to take her out for a drink.*

9. DON'T WEAR A SLEEVELESS OR STRAPLESS DRESS *if the wedding is very conservative or you're not comfortable showing your arms. Otherwise, definitely do!*

10. WEAR A CONSERVATIVE, LIGHT-COLORED SUIT TO ~~AN AFTERNOON CHURCH WEDDING.~~ *a parent-teacher conference. Wear something flirty and feminine to a wedding.*

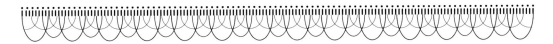

The only rules for a modern-day wedding guest are to keep your cleavage covered and not show up in a floor-length white lace dress, so it's up to you to find the motivation to bring your fashion A-game.

We don't have many chances to get really dressed up these days. A wedding is your chance, so take it. Feel free to throw on that trusty little black dress (or even better, that little red dress, or that little yellow dress) that fits you perfectly, but don't get lazy with your accessories—a lace shawl and bright shoes will step your outfit up a notch. Or try a slim-fitting pantsuit with pearls and a lace camisole. And don't forget a shiny clutch!

As a Bridesmaid

About ten years ago, a miracle occurred. This miracle didn't get much media attention, because the people who run the media are rich old men who are not often invited to be bridesmaids. If women had been in charge of the presses, however, you would have seen articles like the one on the following page.

Thanks to this newfound freedom to choose flattering dresses, most women no longer fear being asked to be bridesmaids. But choosing a becoming bridesmaid dress is not without its challenges. Here are some tips to keep in mind as you shop around:

1. **THE NECKLINE IS THE ABSOLUTE MOST IMPORTANT PART OF THE DRESS.** It frames your face, appears in all the photos, and determines your level of cleavage.

2. **YOU AND YOUR DRESS** are going to be on the photo wall of your friend's house for eternity. Do yourself a favor and take a digital camera with you while dress shopping. Snap some quick pictures of yourself fake walking down the aisle holding flowers, fake standing next the bride, fake dancing with your arms above your head. Review the photos and make sure you look as fabulous in them as you do in the slimming dressing room mirror.

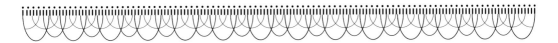

NON-MATCHING BRIDESMAID DRESS TREND
SWEEPS THE NATION

Brides everywhere have stopped trying to fit bridesmaids of all shapes and sizes into the same dress style, opting instead to simply pick a color scheme and allow the wedding party to choose flattering, comfortable dresses on their own. This trend marks a major shift from previous bridesmaid customs, which tended to decimate the self-worth of bridesmaids and/or cause them to never want to see the bride again.

"I just got to thinking," said a bride who agreed to an interview on condition of anonymity, "that maybe my petite friend; my tall, flat-chested friend; and my plus size friend wouldn't appreciate being crammed into the exact same dresses in front of a large crowd and then having their pictures taken." The bride's motives, however, weren't purely selfless. "I still want them to be my friends after the wedding. I need to complain to someone about my husband, right?"

Top scientists have indicated this new practice could have profound consequences. Studies are still being conducted, but researchers at UCLA have already found that allowing bridesmaids to choose their own dresses reduces fidgeting and scowling in wedding photos by up to 80 percent.

3. **CONVENTIONAL WISDOM SAYS BRIDESMAID DRESSES HAVE TO BE UGLY** so even the prettiest gal won't outshine the bride. While this pettiness has (mostly) passed, you still want to make sure you aren't taking away attention from the woman of the day. That means no low-cut strappy numbers, no push-up bras or supertight sheaths, no sequins or fur linings. Think of yourself as a beautiful accessory, but never as the main event.

4. **BEWARE OF THE ALPHA BRIDESMAID (AB).** Even if the laid-back bride has granted you freedom of dress, you might end up in a boob-squashing sheath just because AB wants everyone in the party to wear a different neckline. Stand your ground: if three out of four bridesmaids are in strapless gowns because that style looks best on their bodies, so be it. A happy wedding party is a beautiful wedding party.

Now, even in these liberal modern times, there is a chance you will be assigned a bridesmaid dress. If this happens, try to convince your friend to let you pick out your own shoes and jewelry, and use your accessories to bring in your own (subtle) style. A hippie friend of mine once got stuck wearing a garish purple tulle gown; but when she put on her favorite silver leaf pendant, she suddenly looked natural and comfortable, like she had just thrown on this garish purple tulle gown to pick up some organic rutabagas.

Not to scare the crap out of you or anything, but as a bridesmaid, you will be walking down the aisle and all eyes will be on you. You will be standing in front of a crowd and all eyes will be on you. You will be moving around the reception, greeting crazy old aunts, getting vodka shots for the bride, trying to act cool around her hot older brother, and all eyes will be on you. If your peach satin bridesmaid dress is not doing you any favors, do yourself a favor and get some serious undergarments to smooth you out, hold you in, and prop you up (see Chapter 4 for tips).

STYLE LESSON #44:

If you're a bridesmaid who doesn't get to choose your own dress (the horror!), choose your own shapewear, and choose it well.

Just like summer camp is no place to give your kid a "break" from his meds, a wedding is no time to mess around with an old cotton bra and some shapeless undies. Get yourself a great-fitting bra that works with your dress, Lycra on the hips if needed, control top tights—whatever it takes to make you feel a little more comfortable having all eyes on you.

I Now Pronounce You a Lover of Separates

A couple years ago, Rachel, my best friend since the second grade, called me to say she and her longtime boyfriend Scott, a classmate of mine since the third grade (umm . . . could this story get any cuter?) were getting married. They decided to have the wedding at her house on the Fourth of July, because every year on that day, Rachel's extended family makes a pilgrimage there to blow up massive amounts of illegal fireworks. The bride-to-be thought it would be natural to squeeze in a wedding between the mortar explosions. (This is why Rachel is my best friend.)

As the wedding plans came together, I asked her who was going to officiate at the ceremony. Rachel and Scott are not religious and obviously weren't interested in a traditional wedding. She said, "Oh, damn. Good question."

Now a while back, my younger brother had received a large package in the mail. When I asked him what it was, he opened it, pulled out a Certificate of Ministry, and said, "I'm a reverend, bitch!" Apparently he'd found a Web site that ordains anyone and, for $29.95, sends you a Deluxe Reverend Package that includes, in my brother's words: "A 'Certificate of Ministry' that some guy obviously made at home with Microsoft Publisher, a wallet-sized Reverend ID card that some guy obviously made at home with Microsoft Publisher and a laminator, and a glossy folder with a picture of a rose on the front."

With credentials like those, I couldn't help but offer Rachel my brother's services. We both laughed, knowing my brother hates speaking in front of people (actually hates speaking in general) and would be more than likely to drop a few F-bombs during the ceremony.

Then, one of us joked I should perform the ceremony. We both laughed again, but you know how sometimes, over the course of a conversation, a joke becomes serious? And then all of a sudden you're researching online ordinations that aren't run by a guy in his mom's basement with Microsoft Publisher and a laminating machine? Yeah, that happened.

Within a few days, I was Reverend Winona.

Guests were invited, vows were written, and in what seemed like no time at all, it was late June. Everything was perfect, except I had nothing to wear. I could now legally perform marriages, funerals, last rites, baptisms, and absolve people of their sins, but for the life of me I couldn't find a Reverend Dress.

I went shopping nearly every day, trying on dozens of summery formal dresses, but they were all uncomfortable and unflattering. I've always had a hard time finding dresses that fit me, but this ensemble posed an even greater challenge—I needed a dress that matched my serious responsibility but also my youth and personality, didn't show too much cleavage (nobody likes a wanton reverend), and would be bearable in the 90-degree July heat. I seriously considered wearing my high school graduation gown to perform the ceremony, but Rachel said she'd prefer that I not dress as Gandalf the Wizard.

The day before the wedding, I went to the mall and bought a gorgeous royal blue flared skirt and a black blouse. Under normal circumstances, I would have been thrilled with these purchases, but I felt like a failure. I hadn't found the perfect dress. I hadn't found any dress, actually. In hindsight, and after seeing the pictures, I realize that outfit was more perfect than any dress: I looked like a credible reverend during the vows, but I was comfortable enough to shoot off Roman candles afterward.

STYLE LESSON #45:

Don't forget about separates for special occasions, because sometimes the perfect dress isn't a dress at all.

I think we often get hung up on the idea of the perfect dress, whether it be for a date, a charity gala, or your stint as your best friend's reverend, and we forget separates can be just as formal and a lot more fun to shop for. Try a white button-up blouse with a full, shiny black ball gown skirt for a classic, elegant look, or start with a striking top and find an under-stated skirt for a base. Separates are a great way to create a style of your own when no off-the-rack dress will suffice.

THE #1 SECRET TO LOOKING GOOD AT ANY SPECIAL OCCASION

Whether you're going to a wedding, a blind date, a birthday party at a never-ending pasta buffet, or a humiliating televised smile contest, your outfit is important, and the most important thing about your outfit is that you feel good in it. Take a half step out of your comfort zone in order to create an outfit that's memorable and beautiful, but whether you're wearing denim or diamonds (or both), make sure you feel like you.

TWELVE

Putting It All Together:
GO-TO OUTFITS FOR THE GAL WHO GOES EVERYWHERE

WELL, YOU DID IT! YOU MADE IT THROUGH THE WHOLE BOOK, and I'm proud to bestow upon you the title of *Certified Fashion Expert* (for $15 and a batch of cookies I'll even print you out a little badge!). I hope the previous pages made you laugh, cry (well, in a good way), and get excited to take control of your fashion future.

For one last shot of style inspiration, here are eight complete outfit ideas perfect for a variety of occasions, from spending a Saturday at the park with your best friend to rocking out with an aging-but-awesome band to landing a job that's totally out of your league. These go-to outfits have got you covered. Literally.

YOUR "FELL ASLEEP WATCHING JAPANESE GAME SHOWS AND FORGOT TO DO THE LAUNDRY AND NOW IT'S 6 A.M. AND YOU HAVE NOTHING TO WEAR TO WORK" OUTFIT

STYLE LESSON #46:

Have a flattering, comfortable, professional work outfit on hand—seriously, the full outfit should be hanging up in the back of your closet, ready to grab—for those panicked weekday mornings when you have nothing to wear.

THE ESSENTIALS:

➤ Black pants or skirt with a little stretch
➤ Long sweater in a bright color
➤ Fitted black blazer
➤ Pointy-toe flats

OPTIONAL ADD-ONS:

➤ Tights
➤ Classic trench coat
➤ Fabulous work bag

NOT RECOMMENDED:

➤ Your pajamas

ALSO WORKS FOR:

➤ Facilitating a meeting
➤ Post-work drinks and buffalo wings
➤ Running for political office

Bonus Tip: When you find a work-appropriate piece that you totally love, consider buying two: one for daily wear and one for your emergency backup office outfit.

YOUR "HOSTING A DINNER PARTY TO CELEBRATE YOUR FRIEND GETTING OUT OF A CODEPENDENT RELATIONSHIP" OUTFIT

THE ESSENTIALS:

➤ Simple blouse with pretty details
➤ Flared floral skirt
➤ High heels (you'll take them off after ten minutes)

OPTIONAL ADD-ONS:

➤ Cozy sweater
➤ Long strands of fake pearls
➤ Frilly vintage apron
➤ Fuzzy slippers to replace high heels
   when your feet hurt after ten minutes

NOT RECOMMENDED:

➤ Sweatpants. Please.

ALSO WORKS FOR:

➤ Dinner parties celebrating any occasion
➤ Baking cookies alone while listening to Sinatra
➤ Tea with your grandma
➤ At-home dates

Bonus Tip: If you want to ensure your guests dress up too, I've found adding "or else" to the dress code to be quite helpful.

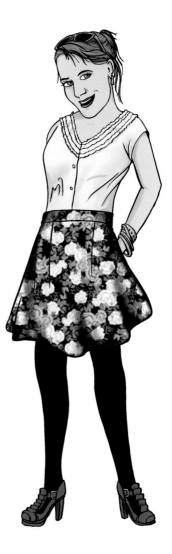

YOUR "MAXED OUT YOUR CREDIT CARD TO SPEND THE WEEKEND IN ROME" OUTFIT

STYLE LESSON #47:

When splurging on spontaneous travel, leave some room in your suitcase and your budget for a pair of killer boots or a couture hat that you can bring home and brag about for years.

THE ESSENTIALS:

➤ Black knee-length jersey skirt (comfy, flattering, and doesn't need to be washed for days)
➤ Light pink slim-fitting V-neck T-shirt
➤ Colorful silk scarf (to hide your tourist pedigree)
➤ Canvas messenger bag
➤ Black flats (for the love of God, anything but sneakers!)

OPTIONAL ADD-ONS:

➤ Lightweight sweater
➤ Dark sunglasses
➤ Glamorous bike shorts (to be worn underneath skirt to prevent thigh chafing)

NOT RECOMMENDED:

➤ "Proud to be an American" T-shirt

ALSO WORKS FOR:

➤ Coffee date with a friend
➤ Lazy Sunday perusing flea markets and bookstores
➤ Summer film festival
➤ Game night

Bonus Tip: There is nothing worse than arriving at your destination with a suitcase full of wrinkled clothes, so bring easy, wrinkle-resistant fabrics. (Actually, arriving at your destination with a suitcase full of clothes covered in toothpaste might be worse, so double-bag all your toiletries, too.)

YOUR "JOB INTERVIEW FOR A JOB YOU'RE NOT QUALIFIED FOR" OUTFIT

STYLE LESSON #48:

A job interview is like a costume party. Come dressed up for the job you want.

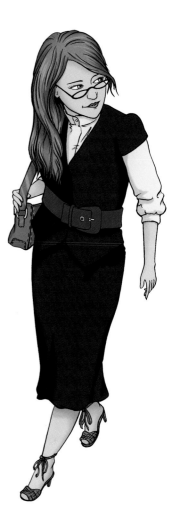

THE ESSENTIALS:

➤ Pencil skirt (if a pencil skirt could talk, it would be eloquent, experienced, and professional, so let it talk for you)
➤ Button-up blouse
➤ Smart little jacket
➤ Satchel or briefcase
➤ A fabulous pair of heels (should be IMMACULATE— nothing kills job interview mojo like scuffed shoes)

OPTIONAL ADD-ONS:

➤ Fabulous belt
➤ Black tights
➤ Delicate wristwatch
➤ Bold glasses

NOT RECOMMENDED:

➤ Glitter eye shadow, resumé printed on pink notebook paper

ALSO WORKS FOR:

➤ Important work presentations
➤ Book club when you didn't read the book
  (you'll look so intimidating, nobody will question you)
➤ Meeting your lover's devoutly religious parents
➤ Sexy secretary fetish

Bonus Tip: A high school friend of mine was once in charge of setting up the chairs at an important event. On his resumé, he listed himself as "Event Chairman." He's now a successful real estate agent.

YOUR "CHARITY DINNER FOR A WILDLIFE PRESERVATION FUND" OUTFIT

STYLE LESSON #49:

No matter how perfect your formal ensemble, drinking one too many mimosas and trying to take a bath in the chocolate fountain will always overshadow your fashion efforts.

THE ESSENTIALS:

➤ Simple-yet-elegant black three-quarter-sleeve blouse (you might have this in your closet right now!)
➤ Blue satin knee-length skirt in a slight bubble shape (separates are easier to shop for)
➤ Zebra print clutch (a subtle nod to the theme)
➤ Gold peep-toe pumps (black would work too)

OPTIONAL ADD-ONS:

➤ Dangly gold or silver earrings
➤ A jeweled hairclip
➤ Lacy hosiery
➤ Shawl or fancy sweater

NOT RECOMMENDED:

➤ Ivory jewelry, mink stole, or snakeskin purse

ALSO WORKS FOR:

➤ Weddings
➤ Fancy gallery openings
➤ High school reunions (*Your high school crush*: "Why are you dressed so fancy? This is a pancake breakfast." *You*: "Oh, I just came from a meeting at the White House.")

Bonus Tip: For formal occasions honoring a specific cause, you're allowed one themed accessory—any more, and you'll be mistaken for the charity's mascot.

YOUR "DAY TRIP TO AN OUTDOOR CONCERT FEATURING AN AGING-BUT-STILL-LEGENDARY CLASSIC ROCK BAND" OUTFIT

THE ESSENTIALS:

➤ Shirtdress
➤ Rugged boots
➤ Cute shoulder bag

OPTIONAL ADD-ONS:

➤ Grandpa sweater
➤ Big sunglasses
➤ Beanie

NOT RECOMMENDED:

➤ High heels

ALSO WORKS FOR:

➤ Summer picnics and barbecues
➤ Book readings
➤ Baseball games
➤ Road trip to the county fair for corn
  dogs and photo opportunities

Bonus Tip: For outdoor events, dress funky and fashionable, but leave anything expensive at home. There's more than a good chance you'll misplace your bag or have an entire beer spilled down your back by a shaky Grateful Dead groupie.

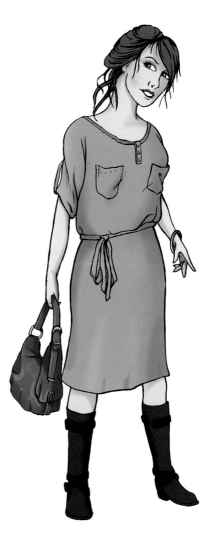

YOUR "SATURDAY AFTERNOON IN THE PARK WITH YOUR BEST FRIEND DISCUSSING THE MEANING OF LIFE" OUTFIT

STYLE LESSON #50:

On casual days, throw on your comfy basics, but bring your whole look together with unique accessories.

THE ESSENTIALS:

➤ Cuffed jeans (perfectly worn-in and a little destroyed = just right!)
➤ Black ribbed tank top
➤ Light brown leather sandals
➤ Bright pink oversized tote bag (the brightly colored tote bag might just be the meaning of life, actually)
➤ Layered gold chain necklaces (adds some interest to a simple, casual outfit)

OPTIONAL ADD-ONS:

➤ Newsboy cap
➤ Aviators
➤ Lightweight jacket in a fun color

NOT RECOMMENDED:

➤ Anything dry-clean only (even if you go to the park in the middle of summer, in the middle of a drought, you are guaranteed to sit in a wet, muddy spot)

ALSO WORKS FOR:

➤ Casual lunch with Mom
➤ Volunteering with kids
➤ Weekend at the beach
➤ Moving day

Bonus Tip: When you are relaxed, casual, and chatting with your best friend, there is a good chance you will meet the love of your life. Look cute.

YOUR "MEETING YOUR ONLINE BOYFRIEND FOR THE FIRST TIME IN A NEUTRAL, PUBLIC PLACE" OUTFIT

THE ESSENTIALS:

➤ Loose button-up shirt
➤ Vest
➤ Cropped pants
➤ Roomy leather bag
➤ Sandals

OPTIONAL ADD-ONS:

➤ Fun bracelets or earrings
➤ Slouchy hat
➤ Pepper spray (hey, you never know)

NOT RECOMMENDED:

➤ Skintight leopard print mini dress

ALSO WORKS FOR:

➤ First day of class at your liberal arts college
➤ Art openings
➤ Late night show at the jazz club
➤ Wine tasting

Bonus Tip: When trying to make a good first impression, people either clam up and dress way too bland or try too hard and overdo it: go for a middle ground that showcases your unique style and keeps you comfortable.

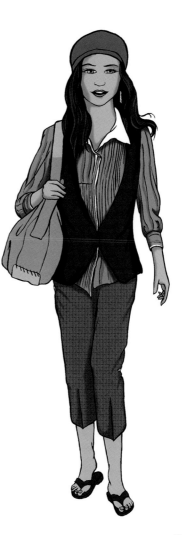

Index

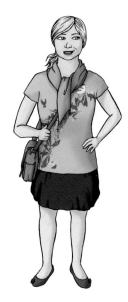

About the Author

Winona Dimeo-Ediger writes the fashion blog Daddy Likey (daddylikey.blogspot.com), which is read in more than 100 countries and has been featured in *Newsday*, *Fashion Week Daily*, and Glamour.com, among other online and print publications. When she is not blogging about cute shoes, she writes for *National Geographic* magazine. Winona splits her time between her apartment in Portland, Oregon, and the sale racks at Nordstrom.

About the Illustrator

Sam Trout is a graphic designer, illustrator, and clothing label based in Seattle who specializes in stylish graphic T-shirts and sweatshirts, examples of which can be seen at www.samtrout.com.
Sam has promoted the Seattle crafter/DIY scene with his event "I Heart Rummage," held fine art shows, and starred as designer, emcee, and model in various fashion shows . . . and as a result has become a recognizable personality in the Seattle art and fashion scenes.